THE RESOURCEFUL PATIENT

J. A. Muir Gray CBE, DSc, MD

eRosetta Press, Oxford, UK

Enquiries should be addressed to:
eRosetta Press at 59 Lakeside, Oxford OX2 8JQ, UK.

The text was written by Muir Gray and the book was
created by Harry Rutter.

The ideas expressed in this book are the personal
vision of the author and do not represent the
views of the Department of Health.

ISBN 1-904202-00-4

Digitally printed in Great Britain by Alden Digital, Oxford
18 February 2002

This book is dedicated to our families.

Muir Gray and Harry Rutter

Acknowledgements

Many of the ideas contained in *The Resourceful Patient* were formed in the course of work that we have done to develop open and honest screening programmes. We are grateful to everyone who helped in its preparation: Amanda Adler, Joan Austoker, Emma Boulton, Iain Chalmers, Kay Chamberlain, Alison Chapple, Andrew Chivers, John Churchill, Jane Collins, Angela Coulter, Tom Delbanco, Ann Dixon-Brown, Anna Donald, Graham Easton, Vicky Entwistle, John Fletcher, Bob Gann, Jackie Gray, Andrew Herxheimer, Alison Hill, Margaret Holmes-Rovner, Tony Hope, Alex Jadad, Lucy Jenkins, Ann McPherson, Henry McQuay, Theresa Marteau, Beth Micklethwaite, Andrew Moore, Al Mulley, Cyril Needham, Annette O'Connor, Sandy Oliver, Mike Parker, Julietta Patnick, John Powell, Steve Pugh, David Rovner, Harriet Rutter, Dave Sackett, Theo Schofield, Sasha Sheppard, Richard Smith, Ann Southwell, Allison Streetly, Thomas Stuttaford, Ben Toth, Pat Ward, Judy Wilson, Jane Wyatt, Sue Ziebland.

Muir Gray and Harry Rutter

Contents

TO THE BOOKMAKERS

Bookmaker:
   A printer and bookbinder. (1515)
   One who compiles or composes a book (often disparagingly). (1533)
   A professional betting-man. (1862)

                              Shorter Oxford English Dictionary

Why the worthy toil of composing or compiling books should ever
have been disparaged by the title 'bookmaker', is not explained in that
treasure house, the *Shorter Oxford English Dictionary*. Publishing, as an
activity distinct from writing and printing, was a term which came
into common use in about 1700. For the last four hundred years,
three distinct trades of writing, printing and publishing were clearly
distinguishable, and the current meaning of the term 'bookmaker'
evolved in the nineteenth century.

The revolution in writing and printing, enabled by new software and
the Web, is transforming the business of making books. At one end
of the chain still sits the author, scribbling in pencil, preferably a 2B,
with the translation to Word effected by the incomparable Rosemary
Lees, his amanuensis for nearly a quarter of a century. About a mil-
lion words have been produced in this way with an editor in the off-
ing, guiding and cajoling, before releasing the 'manuscript' for its
transmutation into a book.

In *The Book Business: Publishing, Past Present and Future* Jason Epstein,
the publishing guru and co-founder of the New York Review of
Books, gives a powerful, clear and realistic vision of a future in which
a single copy of a book, ordered by a reader punching numbers or
typing text into a machine about the size of those that dispense Pepsi
and Coca-Cola, would be rewarded in a few minutes with the clunk
of a book dropping into the receptacle, printed, glued and bound.

Although we are some years away from this position, printing is
changing fast, and a print run of 10 or 25, or 17 or 29 (if that is
the number of people coming to your conference) is no longer
impossibly more expensive than the print run of 2,000 or 3,000 that
high risk monographs such as this one usually merit. Furthermore, a
print run of 10 can be kept on the author's shelf for mailing out as
e-mail orders come in, thus doing away with the pleasureless expense

of lorries, warehouses, stock control, and, all too often, pulping or remaindering. The pleasurable expense of the bookshop, about one-third the price of a book sold there, can also be dispensed with. Bookshops rarely stock those high risk monographs, preferring the perennial sellers like J K Rowling, or the heavily promoted best-sellers by Victoria Beckham or Nigella Lawson.

The first printing of this book was done in three days, from Word file to book in hand; the second printing, with simultaneous production of the e-book version and web site, took less than twenty-four hours. Obviously this required a very clever printer, and The Alden Press in Oxford, a sixth generation company in that city of venerable printers, provided a team who could realise the future – Steve Neville, Brian Jelf, Robert Hay, Jo Wainwright and their visionary and practical Chief Executive, William Alden.

The ability of the printers to produce the book with such speed, however, was due not only to their skill but also to the architecture of the file delivered to them. The production of a hybrid book – paper plus electronic – is the result of the design and building of a document created expressly for this purpose by the book's architect, Harry Rutter. The book architect subsumes the functions of commissioning editor looking after a linear text, but needs to think in four dimensions, creating a hypertext in which every part can be linked to every other part, which will evolve over time.

Finally, thanks are due to Otto Rutter, whose arresting photograph on the cover not only attracts the eye but reminds the reader that the changes we recommend may seem radical to the patient of 2002, but the generation of Otto Rutter, who will be 20 in 2021, will expect the resources we describe to be routinely available, and the culture of clinical practice to be one which starts from the assumption that the patient is in charge.

GENTLE READER

'Gentle Reader' – with these words the 18th and 19th century author would self-consciously remind readers that what they were reading had been written by somebody who wished to guide them through the text. Reading is now so widespread and common, it is assumed that readers will know how to cope with a book and do not need to be told what to expect in the chapter or how to feel about it. In his set of essays on _The Order of Books_, the French writer Roger Chartier emphasises the ephemeral task of the reader and the responsibility that writers felt to guide them through their work. The early authors even gave consideration to the physiology of reading, described by Adrian Johns in _The Nature of the Book_, but most authors now expect readers to be able to plunge into a book, and to use the index, footnotes and references as familiar landmarks in the cartography of reading.

However, this book, although it appears to be a book like any other, such as _The Oxford Textbook of Medicine_, or _Landscape and Memory_ by Simon Schama, is not quite what it appears and therefore, Gentle Reader, we feel a responsibility, which you may find paternalistic, to say a little bit about the book and how it can be read.

Is it a book or a Web site?

The writing of this book was based on a premise unsupported by evidence – the premise being that the creation of a book that was conceived as hypertext could be converted into linear text and vice versa. Linear text is now very familiar, not surprisingly because the earliest written text, the papyrus, was a beautiful example of a linear text (the longest surviving papyrus is about thirty feet long). People are accustomed to writing linear text and the very recent advent of hypertext, namely the ability to order a set of documents not in a long line but in a network, linked using browser software, either on the Web or on a hard disk, is not so familiar and the translation from one to another is often difficult. Our prior assumption was that if we conceived of a text that would be read on the World Wide Web, such a text could both be presented on the Web and also very easily converted into linear text for printing.

This was the initial assumption and much of the text was already written when one of the team asked, 'What is the difference between an e-book and a Web site? Surely it is just a large-scale Web site?'

This gave the writer considerable food for thought, but the answer that eventually emerged was that an electronic book was one that was designed not only to be read in a linear fashion but also, if desired, to be printed out as a book, whereas a Web site was never intended to be printed. We therefore arrived at the decision to create a hybrid book using both electronic means and paper.

Creating an e-book

There has been an explosion of e-books, stimulated by authors such as <u>Stephen King</u>. However, e-books vary in layout, and we propose to create two types of e-book.

The whole of the text will be delivered on the Web, but cut up into small pieces because <u>Jakob Nielsen,</u> one of our gurus, has found that people don't mind clicking but they hate scrolling. We are planning, therefore, Gentle Reader, to make the whole of the book available on the World Wide Web, but in very small gobbets.

We are also making this book available as an e-book, able to be downloaded and read on a hand-held computer.

This is a small example of a long debate in which the e-book concept and the Web site were confused, then distinguished, then confused again, but they are now, if not clarified, at least able to give us a working basis for this, our first attempt to create a hybrid book. The electronic version of the book will in fact be available in two forms – on the Web and as a downloadable e-book.

The hybrid book

In addition to having two electronic versions of the book, we also decided to have a printed version (based on the principle that what distinguished an e-book from a Web site was the ability to print it), and we plan to do this using print-on-demand technology.

Conventional publishing has been hamstrung for many years, particularly in the publishing of monographs, by the agonising consideration given to the length of the print run. With old technology, the set-up costs were so great that it was necessary to have a long print run to justify the printing costs. When, however, you had a long print run, you also had a lot of books, which had to be moved in a lorry to a warehouse, stored, and then re-shipped to the bookshops for as long as the warehouse manager was willing to maintain them. When that point was reached, along came the pulper. If the book was very successful, a second edition would be commissioned, usually after a lapse of several years.

With print-on-demand technology, however, it is possible to change the book every year or every month or every day, and the concept of an edition becomes irrelevant. For this reason, each version or printing of the book is dated, and the date indicates the moment in time at which the last change was made.

The potential of print-on-demand is considerable. If, for example, you have a workshop coming up with seventeen people attending, print-on-demand allows the book to be updated and then for eighteen copies to be printed, seventeen for the delegates and one for the workshop organiser. If, as a result of the workshop, the author wishes to change the book, it can be done simply and electronically, but no more need be printed until the next individual or group places an order.

References and further reading

We have decided to adopt a new approach to references and further reading, making use of new technology.

In the printed book, we have underlined the names of books, the names of authors, and the titles of the articles in the reference section. In addition, certain bits of the text are underlined.

Wherever text is underlined, you can find a Web link on the book's Web site. For example, when we are referring to the book by David Halberstam called *The Best and the Brightest*, David Halberstam is underlined and then *The Best and the Brightest* is underlined. If you read the book beside a computer linked to the Web, you can either find the text on the Web site or look at the book list. The David Halberstam link takes you to an essay on this wonderful writer, the title of the book takes you to the relevant order form in Amazon.

Those bits of the text that are underlined offer you links to other Web sites that we have found which we believe help illuminate the ideas in the book. These Web links will change and grow as we find more resources, but, due to the glory of print-on-demand, each printed version of the book will relate to the Web links given on the Web site. We have not given Web links as URLs because the writer in particular is relatively kack-handed and finds it impossible to translate long URLs from written text to his Internet Explorer bar. We have assumed that the reader of this book would have easy access to the Web, either to look at the Web site while reading the book or to make a note of Web sites to visit later.

The references to articles provide hyperlinks from the Web site of the book either to the wonderful *British Medical Journal* Web site, for it, the paragon of journals, gives access to full text, or, when the references are to articles in other journals, to abstracts provided by PubMed, one of the wonders of modern medicine.

As you like it

We are therefore, Gentle Reader, offering a number of options. You can:

- read the book on your knee or on the train, clutching the familiar paper and turning the familiar page, or

- read the book sitting beside a computer linked to the World Wide Web allowing you to check the references or read in more detail the background evidence to the propositions in the book, or simply explore the Web sites covering concepts or people that stimulate your interest, or

- buy and download the e-book to read on your lap- or hand-held computer using software for reading e-books, or

- roam about the Web site seeing the text, and the links.

Whichever route you choose, Gentle Reader, we hope you find the ideas in the book of interest. The construction of the book has been an adventure for all of us. Undoubtedly we have made mistakes, for we could find no template to follow and no guidebook to the writing of electronic books. In three years' time all of this effort may turn out to be a great mistake because the media may develop in quite different ways and our concept of an e-book may be redundant.

However, we hope that the content of the book will be more relevant in three years' time as the need for a new paradigm in medicine and healthcare is seen to develop.

The 21st century paradigm

Of central importance in this process of transformation is the transformation of the patient's part in healthcare.

The writer of this book is a 57-year-old male. At present, if he were to be admitted to hospital with a myocardial infarction, survive and be discharged, the hospital's primary focus for communication would be his general practitioner, an excellent GP called Dr McPherson. It is recommended by the Department of Health that, in future, the writer should also receive a copy of the letter to Dr McPherson. Dr McPherson will be told that the writer would benefit from aspirin and beta blockers and then an appointment should be arranged with the Cardiology Department. In a year's time Dr McPherson would probably check to ensure that this has been done, and in two years' time she may well be paid according to how well she has done this. This is almost completely impossible to sustain. Surely the writer should be sent a letter by the hospital telling him that he needs aspirin and beta-blockers, and giving him the postal and e-mail addresses for the Cardiology Department, so that he can arrange an appointment? He could be told, of course, that Dr McPherson and the practice nurse would be very pleased to discuss these options with him. He could be told that Dr McPherson would be willing to take over complete management of his care if he feels overwhelmed by the anxiety and responsibility, as some people are, no matter how well-educated.

At present it is assumed that the doctor is the responsible person, and the patient incompetent and in need of care. As the book will argue, this assumption is wrong, and it creates an unsustainable pressure on healthcare professionals. Even if only 10% of patients would like to share decision-making – and the evidence is that the proportion would be much higher in certain age and social groups – the basic premise should be that the patient is competent, not that the patient is incompetent. Even when groups of patients who might be thought to be incompetent are considered, it cannot be assumed that everyone is incompetent. Furthermore, even though only a minority of patients wish full control or shared decision-making, the majority of patients would like more information and involvement than they get at present.

This book is committed to promoting the concept of the resourceful patient, namely the patient who is not only aware of his rights but is also made aware of his responsibilities and is willing to accept them, provided, of course, that he is given the resources to do so.

The book is in four parts:

- the first describes the rise and fall of the medical empire;

- the second part describes what doctors do all day, because a failure to understand this often leads to confusion and conflict;

- the third part describes the resources that patients need in order to share responsibility and assume more control;

- the fourth part describes the patients, clinicians and organisations of the 21st century when the new paradigm is in place.

Gentle Reader, read on.

Section 1

The Rise and Fall of the Medical Empire – the Evolution of Medical Power

The Pulitzer Prize for 1984 was awarded to <u>Paul Starr</u> for his monumental study of <u>*The Social Transformation of American Medicine*</u>, sub-titled 'The Rise of a Sovereign Profession and the Making of a Vast Industry'. The book is divided into two parts: the first tracing 'the rise of medical authority' from the 18th century to 1930; the second heralding the coming of the corporation, and describing the impact that the corporation and the growing role of the State had on medical authority.

Recent discussions in the United Kingdom have focused on the need to empower patients, and the arguments sometimes appear to indicate that the medical profession has been omnipotent for ever. However, this has not been the case, and what we have seen in the last hundred years has been the rise (and, more recently, the decline) of medical power and, consequently, a decline (and then, more recently, a resurgence) in patient power.

This book is in four parts. This first part charts the waxing and waning of medical power and is set out in the following chapters.

1.1 A resourceful patient
1.2 The shifting balance of power
1.3 The four dimensions of medical decline
1.4 The decline in sapiential authority
1.5 The decline of moral authority
1.6 The decline in bureaucratic authority
1.7 The decline in charismatic authority

1.1 A resourceful patient

It was to be the consultant physician's last visit and Dalgliesh suspected that neither of them regretted it – arrogance and patronage on one side and weakness, gratitude and dependence on the other being no foun-

dation for a satisfactory adult relationship however transitory. He came into Dalgliesh's small hospital room preceded by Sister, attended by his acolytes, already dressed for the fashionable wedding which he was to grace as a guest later that morning. He could have been the bridegroom except that he sported a red rose instead of the customary carnation. Both he and the flower looked as if they had been brought and burnished to a peak of artificial perfection, gift-wrapped in invisible foil, and immune to the chance winds, frosts and ungentle fingers which could mar more vulnerable perfections. As a final touch, he and the flower had both been lightly sprayed with an expensive scent, presumably an aftershave lotion. Dalgliesh could detect it above the hospital smell of cabbage and ether to which his nose had become so inured during the past weeks that it now hardly registered on the senses. The attendant medical students grouped themselves round the bed. With their long hair and short white coats they looked like a gaggle of slightly disreputable bridesmaids.

Dalgliesh was stripped by Sister's skilled impersonal hands for yet another examination. The stethoscope moved, a cold disc, over his chest and back. This last examination was a formality but the physician was, as always, thorough; nothing he did was perfunctory. If, on this occasion, his original diagnosis had been wrong, his self-esteem was too secure for him to feel the need for more than a token excuse. He straightened up and said:

'We've had the most recent path. report and I think we can be certain now that we've got it right. The cytology was always obscure, of course, and the diagnosis was complicated by the pneumonia. But it isn't acute leukaemia, it isn't any type of leukaemia. What you're recovering from — happily — is an atypical mononucleosis. I congratulate you, Commander. You had us worried.'

'I have you interested; you had me worried. When can I leave here?'

P.D. James, The Black Tower

Toughened by the death of his wife and son, not to mention the exigencies of his gruesome job, Adam Dalgliesh must have developed competence, resilience and confidence to a degree that few other patients could match. Few of us would have the resolve or speed of thought to respond to the consultant physician's patronising statement so trenchantly. Even such a powerful personality as Dalgliesh would, however, have made little permanent impact on the confident carapace of the consultant who would continue to dominate his consultations, although even he, one suspects, would in future probably be more circumspect about his phrase 'you had us worried'.

Fortunately, the description of the consultation seems dated, even for the publication date – 1975, a throwback perhaps to the 1950s when the consultant, especially in a London teaching hospital, exuded power, and the patient was submissive and subservient.

The very word 'patient' has two definitions in the *Shorter English Dictionary*, namely: 'one who is under medical treatment' and 'one who suffers patiently' or 'a person … to whom something is done', but there is no need for a person who is suffering to be powerless, and the shift of power from patient to physician occurred relatively recently, during the second half of the twentieth century. In the first decades of the 21st century, the balance of power will shift back from physicians and clinicians to patients, as the benefits of patient empowerment become clear.

1.2 The shifting balance of power

Doctors were not always powerful. In the 19th century their social status was low, lower than that of the clergy or the legal profession. They were, of course, able to have a reasonable social status, but only if they were well connected, as was Mr Lydgate, the surgeon in George Eliot's *Middlemarch*, who was 'one of the Lydgates of Northumberland, really well connected', although, as Lady Chettam pointed out, 'one does not expect it in a practitioner of that kind. For my own part I like a medical man more on the footing of a servant, they are often all the cleverer'. *Middlemarch* (now available in its entirety online, thanks to the wonderful Gutenberg Project) was published in 1871, and describes perhaps better than any other book the ambivalent, but rising, status of the doctor in Britain during its first phase of modernisation.

1.2.1 In the 19th century, patients had more power

Jane Austen's *Emma* was written more than fifty years earlier in 1816, and describes the hypochondriacal Mr Woodhouse making use of the apothecary, Perry, who was clearly the social inferior of the valetudinarian. Between 1820 and 1870, the social position of the doctor had begun to improve, partly because, as a result of the railway revolution which started about 1850, even rural England was in the process of rapid change by 1870. Science and technology were in the ascendant and the Church, although not yet in decline, was being challenged as never before by new wealth and new ideas.

1.2.2 By the end of the 20th century, physicians had more power

At which point in time did the balance of power swing from patient to doctor? There is no specific answer to this question, but it occurred after the Second World War when scientific medicine was starting to have an impact. Science alone, however, is only one factor in determining the relative balance between doctor and patient.

What factors affect the power balance between clinician and patient? Obviously there are many, and generalisations are fraught with difficulties, but there are a few obvious determinants of where the power lies.

Knowledge. As science provided more knowledge for clinicians, their authority increased – what sociologists call 'sapiential authority'. This is not to say that patients gave up their beliefs, but they certainly deferred overtly to the power of authority of the doctor, even though his science was often flawed, as beautifully depicted in J. G. Farrell's book _The Siege of Krishnapur_.

The changing financial contract between clinician and patient. Until the advent of the National Health Service, patients really were consumers or customers and shopped around, if they could afford it. The provision of services by the State, which removed the financial dependence of the doctor on the patient, was undoubtedly a relief to many patients, but it did shift the balance of power towards the clinicians, particularly as the clinician was virtually a monopoly supplier of medical care to patients who had, in the United Kingdom at least, great difficulty in changing the general practitioner on whose list they had been placed.

The rise of the meritocracy. During the second half of the twentieth century Britain experienced what the sociologist Michael Young called 'the rise of the meritocracy', and the medical profession, like other knowledge-based professions, became more powerful and more respected. Doctors acquired more authority, derived not only from their public commitment to medical self-regulation and high standards, but also from their self-avowed claim to act always and only in the patient's best interests.

1.2.3 All professions are losing power in the 21st century

It is not just medicine that is losing power. _The Death of the Guilds_ is the title of a monumental work by Elliott Krause in which he studied the decline in power of a number of professions, including medicine, in the United States, France, Germany, Italy and the United Kingdom. The subtitle of the book is 'The state capitalism, and the decline of the professions, 1930 to the present day' and Krause demonstrates that even while doctors were increasing their power to control disease, which understandably increased the awe in which they were held by many patients, the medical profession as a whole was losing autonomy and its powers of self-determination and self-regulation. The decline of the power of the medical profession was occurring while the clinical power of the individual doctor was waxing.

Obviously these generalisations do not take into account variations between different groups within society, for example different ethnic groups or the differences between men and women. Nor do they take into account individual factors relating to both the doctor and the patient, for there is a wide range of different styles within all of the groups mentioned above.

1.3 The four dimensions of medical decline

The brooding power of Max Weber dominated sociology for most of the twentieth century, and rightly so. Weber's writing is dense and sometimes difficult, even when translated into English, but the clarity of thought and analysis requires no sociological training for its appreciation; experience of life is sufficient to endorse at least some of Weber's theories, notably his theory on authority. Weber, and several other twentieth century sociologists who followed, identified a number of different types of authority:

- moral;
- bureaucratic;
- sapiential;
- charismatic.

Medical authority has declined in all four of those domains, and the range of powers which doctors have had for a few decades in the twentieth century is also waning. This trend is, perhaps surprisingly, neither lamented by all clinicians nor welcomed by all patients, some of whom might wish to continue to believe that their doctor was omniscient.

1.4 The decline in sapiential authority

Sapiential authority is that which derives from knowledge. As the knowledge base of medicine grew, so too did the authority of doctors. However, although the knowledge base continues to grow dramatically, the sapiential authority of doctors is declining.

1.4.1 Patients are now willing to question doctors

Consumerism is a major trend in all developed countries, and as a result consumers, including patients, are less willing to accept the authority of clinicians.

The term 'consumerism' has now fallen somewhat into disrepute, being regarded as synonymous with conspicuous consumption and the excessive use of the world's resources, and there are Web sites devoted to 'anti-consumerism'. The effects of consumerism, however, are widespread, powerful and, in the main, beneficial.

Thus, although some patients were always more intelligent and better educated than some clinicians, it is only recently that patients have found the confidence to challenge clinicians. Furthermore, patients, or at least their representatives, are now being given tools to question intelligently the propositions and assertions of clinicians, thus increasing their sapiential authority. One of the most important tools that they have been given is the skill of critical appraisal.

The Critical Appraisal Skills Programme (CASP) in the Institute of Health Sciences in Oxford has been designed to give patients and the public both the skills to appraise an article and, even more important, the confidence to ask a clinician in a non-threatening way the simple question: 'How good is the evidence?'

In the CASP Programme, participants are taught how to identify the type of research method that is most appropriate to answer a particular question, and then to appraise articles describing research done using that method to assess the quality of research and therefore the strength of evidence.

As one Board member of a Health Authority said:

'I was really excited when I came to join the Health Authority but as soon as they discovered that I was in property, they put me in charge of the Property Committee and I did the same thing for the Health

Authority as I did in my day job. The CASP Programme is wonderful — it has given me the skills and confidence to ask clinicians some simple basic questions; this is what I joined the Health Authority to do.'

1.4.2 The World Wide Web gives consumers new powers

Patients now have easy access to high quality knowledge.

The sapiential authority of the clinician could be maintained as long as patients were excluded from medical libraries, as was generally the case except in very enlightened settings such as the <u>National Library of Medicine</u> in Washington.

The volume of medical knowledge available to doctors is growing at an exponential rate. One estimate made by <u>Professor David Sackett</u>, when Director of the <u>Centre for Evidence-Based Medicine</u> at the University of Oxford, was that to stay up to date, a general physician would need to read 19 papers every day. It is therefore plainly impossible for any clinician, except the super-specialist, to know everything there is to know, and keep up to date. However, a patient with only a single health problem can keep up to date. For rare diseases the patient may know more than the clinician — except, of course, the clinician in highly specialised centres which patients attend from time to time.

Many patients are better educated than clinicians, and even though the doctor may have a better esoteric knowledge at the start of a patient's journey, the patient can soon overtake the clinician. <u>Stephen Jay Gould</u>, the famous palaeontologist and baseball fan, gives a dramatic description of his acquisition of knowledge, with heartening results:

> *In July 1982, I learned that I was suffering from abdominal mesothelioma, a rare and serious cancer usually associated with exposure to asbestos. When I revived after surgery, I asked my first question of my doctor and chemotherapist: 'What is the best technical literature about mesothelioma?' She replied, with a touch of diplomacy (the only departure she has ever made from direct frankness), that the medical literature contained nothing really worth reading.*

> *Of course, trying to keep an intellectual away from literature works about as well as recommending chastity to Homo Sapiens, the sexiest primate of all. As soon as I could walk, I made a beeline for Harvard's Countway medical library and punched mesothelioma into the computer's bibliographic search program. An hour later, surrounded by the*

latest literature on abdominal mesothelioma, I realised with a gulp why my doctor had offered that humane advice. The literature couldn't have been more brutally clear: mesothelioma is incurable, with a median mortality of only 8 months after discovery. I sat stunned for about 15 minutes, then smiled and said to myself: so that's why they didn't give me anything to read. Then my mind started to work again, thank goodness...

The problem may be briefly stated: what does 'median mortality of 8 months' signify in our vernacular? I suspect that most people, without training in statistics, would read such a statement as 'I will probably be dead in 8 months' – the very conclusion that must be avoided, both because this formulation is false and because attitude matters so much.'

Stephen Jay Gould, 'The median isn't the message' in Adam's Navel

Gould was not trained as a physician but medical knowledge is relatively easy to understand compared, for example, to Arabic and Astrophysics, and an intelligent patient focusing on one disease, can soon become familiar with its concepts, terminology and evidence.

Some clinicians recognise this and argue that, if they want, patients should be given all the knowledge that is available. Anthony Horan, writing in the July 2000 *Newsletter of the American Urological Association*, suggests that urologists

'... tell our patients with incidentally discovered, asymptomatic, low and middle grade prostate and kidney cancers that they have a 50-year-old cancer that, if it kills them, will kill them in about 17 years. If it can metastasize, it has already had 35 years to do it. This changes completely the sense of hurry that pervades cancer counselling. The media speak of cancer as though it were a grenade that quickly gets to a certain size and then explodes. Under the age of tumors proposal, there is time for fourth and fifth opinions.

'We should also inform them of our estimate, based on published doubling times and mean time to death figures, of the time to cancer caused death. We should inform them of their life expectancies as determined by actuaries. Patients and urologists can elect a management strategy based on harmony among the age of the tumor, the predicted mean time to death and the actuarial life expectancy.'

Some patients are already experts; with the correct approach many more could develop expertise, since much of the science of medicine is easily understandable.

1.4.3 Doctors are now willing to say 'I don't know'

What are clinicians to do, faced with patients who come in with a stack of print-out from the World Wide Web, sometimes called 'Le maladie du grand print-out' – a 21st century version of the patronising 20th century term, 'La maladie du petit papier', used to describe patients who presented with some questions written on a bit of paper? The only course for the clinician to follow, bearing in mind the motto of the Chindits that the boldest measures are the safest, is, instead of pretending to know or be up to date, simply to say the three most important words for clinicians in the knowledge era – 'I don't know'.

Surprisingly, although clinicians may find them difficult to say, many patients find them relatively easy to accept, understand and appreciate, and paradoxically it may be that the best way for the clinician to maintain sapiential authority is to disclaim it, providing of course they have the skills to act as a knowledge manager during the consultation.

1.4.4 There is now better knowledge about the frailties of doctors

Patients have not only had better access to knowledge about disease, they also have better knowledge about doctors, and their professed role as honest, disinterested purveyors of scientific information for patients is no longer trusted. With this type of knowledge, public respect for the morality of medicine has been undermined.

1.5   The decline of moral authority

The cynical view of society is that power rests solely with those bold enough or rich enough to seize it, but in the 21st century moral authority is still important. The schoolteacher is still regarded as more of an authority within society than, for example, the bookmaker, even though the income of the latter may be five, ten or twenty times that of the former. This authority derives in part from the moral position of the schoolteacher in society, with the generally held view that teachers are engaged in a task which is seen as having a morally justifiable dimension, namely the guidance of the young.

The moral authority acquired by clinicians in the 20th century has declined in recent years.

Patients now also have much clearer legal rights. The European Convention on Human Rights was adopted by the United Kingdom when the Human Rights Act became law in 1998. The Act came fully into force on 2 October 2000. The European Convention gives the patient the legal right to refuse treatment and, perhaps more significant, consultation with parents and, if necessary, other family members is now legally required, although parents do not necessarily have the last word. A court rules against the parents if it believes that the parents are not acting in the best interests of the child, because the child has also been given greater legal rights by the European Convention.

1.5.1 Doctors are seen to be ordinary mortals – good and bad

The rules governing the medical profession list among the gravest of misdemeanours a sexual relationship with a patient because of the power that a doctor holds, and the possibility of misusing this, to take sexual advantage of a patient. In more recent years, other moral misdemeanours of doctors have received publicity and perhaps the financial shenanigans of doctors who defraud healthcare systems do as much to reduce the moral authority of the medical profession as does sexual indiscretion in these more sexually liberated days. Furthermore, revelations about doctors whose actions have harmed or killed patients, whether for gain, as in the case of Harold Shipman, or because of incompetence, as in the Bristol heart surgery cases, have damaged the moral authority of the profession by shaking public confidence in self-regulation, a cornerstone of the claim that a profession makes to be morally detached from other trades.

The medical profession has suffered a decline in its moral authority, however, not only as a result of changes in public attitudes towards the profession, but as a result of general changes in society's attitudes to science.

1.5.2 The end of the honeymoon with science

For most of the 20th century, science was viewed as an unalloyed good because the Second World War created the power base of science.

For the first time, war was won not by the bravest soldiers or the cleverest generals but by the best scientists, and in the years following the Second World War, science grew in power because of the authority granted to it by society, which accepted the view that science had a moral purpose of creating a better society.

The Manhattan Project, which led to the development of the atom bomb, had shown clearly how science could focus on a major problem and solve it, although even at that time there were doubts about the moral wisdom of using science for this purpose. Nevertheless, for the next twenty years, science was in the ascendant, turning its attention to problems such as cancer and starvation, and producing solutions which were generally regarded as good by society. In the 1960s, however, all this began to change, as a number of people began to describe the down side of science. Some of the key events and trends were:

- thalidomide – the negative side of medical breakthroughs;

- the Vietnam War – the misuse of science to solve a moral and political problem;

- *Silent Spring* – the ecological harm of science.

For readers who want to get a feeling of the heady excitement of the days when science, including the social sciences, were thought to be the solution to every problem from cancer to urban poverty, the best read is David Halberstam's wonderful book *The Best and the Brightest*, which describes the hubris of science and the belief that human beings could solve any problem with its help, epitomised by the excitement of the election of John F. Kennedy to the American Presidency. Kennedy was assassinated before the Vietnam policy demonstrated the impotence of science, when the world's most powerful army failed to overcome a committed people and an army of poorly equipped men using bicycles. The Kennedy years were the honeymoon period in the relationship between science and society.

1.5.3 Fear of a scientific conspiracy

Many people now think that scientists are in league with industry. If science has simply got it wrong, the public could forgive it, but in the 1960s concern started to be expressed about the possibility that science was misusing the trust invested in it by society by conspiring with government and big business to advance its cause, not solely for the good of society, but also for the good of the scientists. The first description of the inter-dependence of science, government and big business came not from an analysis of medical science but from a study of the relationship between science and the defence industry provided by John Kenneth Galbraith, who was both one of Kennedy's closest advisers, and also one of the most perceptive and trenchant critics of the Kennedy hubris of the early 1960s. Galbraith was not only a leading economist, he was also that very rare type of academic – wonderfully readable. His book *The New Industrial Estate*, published in 1967, described an alliance between what he called the military industrial complex, as follows:

Scientists working on defence R&D contracts advise

- generals and admirals who make decisions for

- politicians to take which increase investment in defence and give contracts to

- defence industries which give

  - scientists research contracts and

  - political parties donations and

  - generals jobs when they retire.

The extension of this argument to biological sciences was made by Ulrich Beck in his famous book *The Risk Society*, or, in the original German, *Risikogesellschaft*. In this book Beck, Professor of Sociology at the Ludwig Maximillian University in Munich, observes that science and scientists have thrown in their lot with capitalists and politicians, and as a consequence so-called safe levels of, say, pesticides, are in fact simply a means of licensed poisoning.

1.5.4 The remoralising of medicine

The decline of moral authority provides a strong foundation for the development of a moral basis for clinical practice, to replace the specious authority with which medicine was invested in times past. Instead of assuming moral authority, the 21st century clinician recognises that responsibility has a moral dimension. The clinician who strays from technical to moral decision-making must act with responsibility and not simply shoot from the moral hip.

20th century clinicians made moral decisions on the basis of their personal beliefs and values. Ethics was regarded as a subject which had a bearing on only a few types of clinical decision, notably abortion, euthanasia, and research. The need for research ethics committees was recognised more than thirty years ago but in the 21st century, the dramatic development is that of the clinical ethics committee. The need for such committees arose from the greater awareness among clinicians that they face many moral dilemmas.

Consider the case of Mrs N, a young woman with AIDS in the Intensive Care Unit of the San Francisco General Hospital, as described by John F. Murray in his *Intensive Care: a Doctor's Journal*. The problem was that:

> To the doctors who talked to her at the beginning of this hospitalization, she made her views unmistakably clear: 'I've had AIDS for a long time, but my family don't know about it, and I don't want them to know about it now.' I am quite sure she is going to die, but if she instructed us to be aggressive, we might prolong her life a few weeks and get her back on treatment. At this point, though, we cannot find out what she wants because she is too sick and sedated to tell us.

Because of this commitment he had to seek advice and reports that:

> I met with the chairman of our hospital's Ethics Committee, Dr. Richard Broderick to discuss my concerns about her. We desperately want guidance in determining what we should do if, as seems inevitable, her condition deteriorates. Should we insert more chest tubes if her other lung collapses? Should we use medications to support her blood pressure if it drops? Should we pound on her chest and shock her heart if it stops beating? These are all real prospects. I can't stop thinking about how she's only nineteen years old. Would even a few more weeks of life mean something to her?

> 'We have another tough one', I told him. 'A young woman with AIDS who is steadily losing ground and will probably die soon. We need to decide how aggressive to be. But she's in no shape to tell us, and she told everyone at the beginning of this hospitalization not to discuss matters with her family because she doesn't want them to know she has AIDS. There was and perhaps still is a Mr N, but he abandoned her and vanished a few months after their marriage. I'd like to talk to her father to try to find out if he had any indication about how she wants to be treated. But she has clearly said not to. What do we do now?'

> Today, Dr. Broderick comes to the ICU to tell us that he has thought about our predicament and talked to others on his committee. Their

13

> conclusion is that, despite her explicit interdiction, we can disclose the fact that she has AIDS to her father. To serve as her surrogate and advise us medically on her behalf, he must be informed of the exact situation.
>
> I see the logic, but I am uneasy with this decision because of its contradiction of Mrs N's stated wishes.

Influenced by the Ethics Committee, he proceeds to inform the family with great reservations:

> Full of remorse, I break the news. No one expresses shock or surprise. Her father says, 'Yeah, we know that. She's had it a long time. But she didn't want us to know, so we didn't talk about it.'

These moral dilemmas have always been present in medicine: now they are recognised and managed more responsibly.

The decline of traditional moral authority has been complemented by the development of more thoughtful moral responsibility by clinicians and this provides a much more stable foundation for the resourceful patient who wishes to take decisions, and manage their care.

1.6 The decline in bureaucratic authority

Bureaucratic power is one of the few types of power held by people, not as a result of their wealth, as in a plutocracy, or their birth, as in an aristocracy, or because of popular mandate, as in a democracy, but because of their position within an organisation. Doctors and other clinicians have had bureaucratic authority to complement their moral, sapiential and charismatic authority.

1.6.1 Professional self-regulation was set up in the 19th century

Sarah Gamp, the famous nurse in _Martin Chuzzlewit_ by Charles Dickens, whose sole source of evidence was the imaginary Mrs Harris, could have practised in the United Kingdom until 1902, for it was only then that the Midwives Act was put on the Statute Book, setting up a professional body to regulate them, as the doctors had been regulated earlier by the Medical Act. Doctors had always had some vague accountability, but with the passing of an Act of Parliament doctors were clearly part of a line management system, albeit an imperfect one (Figure 1).

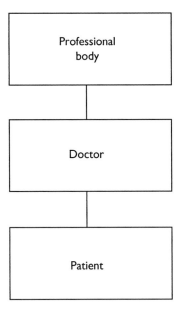

Figure I

1.6.2 Professional self-regulation fell into disrepute in the 20th century

<u>George Bernard Shaw</u> called a profession 'a conspiracy upon the public', and the medical profession came in for an excoriating attack in the preface to <u>*The Doctor's Dilemma*</u>. Although *The Doctor's Dilemma* focused primarily on the financial drivers of medical decision-making, Shaw also wished to highlight the fact that doctors regarded themselves as accountable to no-one but God, a bureaucratic line with the apparatus of professional regulation being regarded as ineffective in managing clinical innovation or clinical competence. For some doctors, particularly hospital consultants, the criticism was taken even further, and in the year 2000, criticisms of hospital doctors were expressed by saying that hospital consultants considered themselves little gods, i.e. accountable to no-one, as shown in Figure 2.

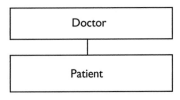

Figure 2

This situation was unacceptable in the age of consumerism, and two types of bureaucratic controls were introduced:

● controls to improve quality and prevent errors;

● cost control measures.

1.6.3 *External regulation has been introduced to supplement self-regulation*

In all countries doctors are increasingly held to account as a result either of court action or a formal complaint. New organisational links are thus set up between the doctor and organisations other than their professional body, as shown in Figure 3.

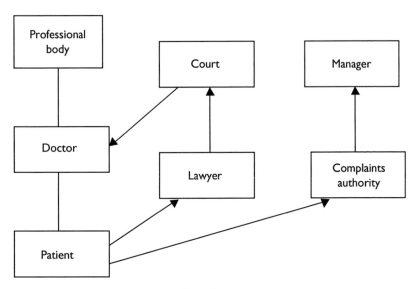

Figure 3

This bureaucratic weight did not increase the authority of doctors. On the contrary, it reduced their authority because patients saw that clinicians had decreased individual power.

1.6.4   External regulation of clinical quality – clinical governance is now in place

In Figure 3, there is no straight line between the manager and the doctor because the relationship between manager and doctor was unclear.

When complaints referred to something to do with the doctor's social conduct – their politeness, for example, the manager could take action, but the doctor's clinical performance was left either to the courts or to the professional bodies to deal with. In 1999, this changed with the introduction of the concept of clinical governance, which now puts a clear line from the manager to the doctor, covering not only the doctor's social graces but also their clinical competence (Figure 4).

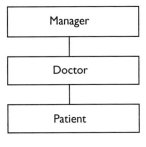

Figure 4

1.6.5 Additional regulation to control costs tightens the screw on professionals

The fate of Sisyphus was to push a large boulder uphill; even worse, as soon as the boulder reached the top it would roll back down again. *Sisyphus or Pegasus*[1] is the title of an article in a prominent American medical journal describing the rapid fall from grace of the American medical profession. The image of Pegasus soaring free and unfettered epitomises the American medical profession in its golden days when budgets were booming and a surgeon could simply put up a shingle in a new town and start to ply for trade. As healthcare became increasingly expensive, the middle classes, an important driving force in American healthcare, began to insure against illness, which had become one of the common causes of personal bankruptcy. The insurance companies, who paid for healthcare, were a new force on the American healthcare scene, and insurance companies began to control cost to maximise return for investors as if they were private companies, as many were.

In the early days of the doctor as Pegasus, the relationship between patient, doctor, diagnosis and treatment was simple (Figure 5).

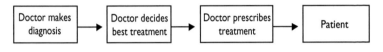

Figure 5

However, diagnostic and treatment guidelines were increasingly introduced, in part by professional bodies keen to reduce the number of court cases and complaints against clinicians, but increasingly by the companies who ultimately paid for treatment. Thus the individual judgement of the doctor was more often tempered by guidelines. Doctors are, however, notoriously difficult to instruct, and com–pliance with guidelines was shown to be limited. Insurance companies, or health maintenance organisations pressed by insurance companies, began to introduce a compulsory second opinion, illustrated in Figure 6.

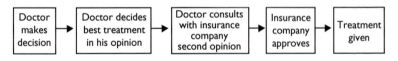

Figure 6

With the compulsory second opinion, the doctor seeing the patient had to phone another doctor or, even worse for some clinicians, a nurse employed by the organisation paying for the healthcare, and check through the treatment decision with them. Sometimes a treatment would be refused, and the doctor would have to explain this to the patient. Jerome Groopman describes these conflicts beautifully in his account of his battle with an insurance company in 'The lottery' (in *Second Opinions*).

1.6.6 Cost control can compromise healthcare providers and clinicians

Partly as a result of the huge payments made to the chief executives of private insurance companies and health maintenance organisations, public anger towards these organisations has grown steadily in the United States, and in the film and book *The Rainmaker*, by John Grisham, the insurance company which had refused treatment to a patient on the grounds of cost, using the excuse of ineffectiveness, was the villain. For some doctors the imposition by payers of guidelines which could be harmful to patients has been the last straw, adding to their bureaucratic burden and reducing their bureaucratic authority (Figure 7).

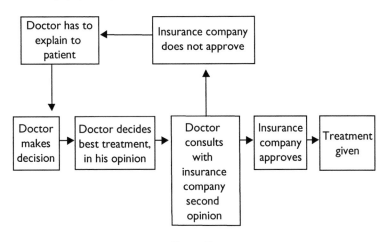

Figure 7

1.6.7 Declining bureaucratic power, increasing administrative burden

Paradoxically, the decline in the bureaucratic power of doctors has been accompanied by an increase in their administrative workload. In 2001, general practitioners in Britain complained about the fact that they often had an hour or two of administrative work every day, much more than was customary a decade earlier, and still had no more clinical time with their patients, whose needs and demands, increasingly more complex and detailed, were being met in consultations which averaged less than ten minutes.

It is good that the bureaucratic power of the doctor has been reduced, but it cannot be good that so much of the time that could be spent with patients is consumed by administration.

The decline in moral, sapiential, and bureaucratic authority of the doctor has reduced their status. Now that the doctor is no longer remote and mysterious, the charismatic authority deriving from that remoteness and mystery is diminished.

1.7 The decline in charismatic authority

Medical power has declined in all four dimensions – moral, bureaucratic, sapiential and charismatic – the last of these being the most subtle but perhaps the most important.

1.7.1 The gift of grace

Charisma, or charism as it is cited in the Shorter English Dictionary, means 'a favour specially vouchsafed by God; a grace; a talent'. Although the term 'charismatic' is sometimes used now as a synonym for an attractive personality, the original meaning applies, or applied, very well to the medical profession, who were seen as healers in society. Before science, healing was a gift of God and Jesus as a healer was considered to have a special gift from God. The doctor as healer, of course, implied that it was the doctor himself (for in those days all were male) who had the healing power, either given by God or deriving from some other source. The work of <u>Michael Balint</u>, which revealed the power of what he called 'the drug doctor', emphasised the importance of the doctor as healer. The <u>Balint Groups</u> of the 1950s did not, however, claim that the power of the doctor was a gift of God. They recognised that it derived in part from the doctor's personality but that it also reflected the faith invested in the clinician by the patient.

1.7.2 The doctor replaced the priest in many communities

The secularisation of western society resulted in a fall from grace of priests. Secularisation is not simply the result of increasing faith in science – other factors, such as increasing population mobility, play a part. What is certain, however, is the decline in charismatic authority of the parish priest, hitherto a figure of central importance throughout the United Kingdom. In the middle of the 19th century the parish priest clearly had more authority than the doctor; by the middle of the 20th century the positions had reversed, although it is hard to determine precisely when the crossing point was reached.

Some doctors complained about this, aware of the fact that they were being brought many problems that would previously have been taken to the parish priest, either because of their moral dimension or because the Church had traditionally managed many problems of unhappiness, which, either presenting directly as depression or presenting in some physical guise, are now taken to the doctor.

1.7.3 Idealistic medical drama inflated the charisma of the medical profession

In the 1950s, A.J. Cronin was a doctor, a graduate of Glasgow University, who achieved fame with a number of novels that had a strong social message, for example *Hatter's Castle*. Cronin's fame today, however, is based largely on the television series, *Dr Finlay's Casebook*, which ran from 1959 to 1966, with a new adaptation in 1993. These stories, set in Callendar in Scotland, gave an idealised picture of a dedicated young doctor interacting with his more cynical older colleague, Dr Cameron. Also in 1959 the television series *Doctor Kildare* was launched, in which the young Richard Chamberlain appeared as an idealised perfect young clinician, again often in conflict with a curmudgeonly older colleague.

1.7.4 Realistic medical drama decreases charisma

Many idealised images of society were portrayed on television in the late 1950s and early 1960s, reflecting the more confident mood in society and the wishes of the media to provide people with escape from the pressures of daily life. Currently-televised medical dramas, for example *Casualty* and *ER*, are much grittier and more realistic, characterised by:

- doctors expressing doubts about their mission;
- nurses challenging doctors;
- ungrateful patients, and;
- doctors revealing the human side of their own lives.

These programmes demythologise the healing professions, and by reducing the myths reduce the charisma, a process accelerated by the medical profession itself.

1.7.5 Medicine is demystifying itself

Both the medical profession as a whole, and individual practitioners to a greater or lesser degree, have become more open, following to some extent the general social trend towards informality and openness.

Three manifestations of this are:

- the clinicians' mode of dress;

- their consulting style; and

- their mode of address to patients.

1.7.5.1 Clinicians' mode of dress

In the 19th century, medicine and nursing were dirty businesses, and special dress was needed. Furthermore, it was recognised that it was often necessary to change one's dress after leaving clinical work for both health and aesthetic reasons. As suppurating infections have become less common and disease less often presents at an advanced stage, clinical care has become less dirty, but until the end of the twentieth century clinicians continued to wear the uniforms which were put on and taken off at either end of the working day, like priestly raiment before and after religious services.

In most hospitals, the nurse's cap, which has become progressively less utilitarian and more symbolic, has now been done away with, and nursing clothes are now much less formal in their appearance than the traditional uniform, which was closer to that of the French maid than to that of a technocrat. The sexual connotations of nursing uniforms, of course, also probably accelerated their demise.

For the doctor the white coat represents, among other things:

- a barrier against infection, its scientific justification;

- a means of identification, its moral justification;

- the healer's pure white mantle, its symbolic justification.

For many doctors a white coat is justifiable, both keeping their own clothes clean and providing a reassuring barrier between the doctor's clothes and the patient. However, white coats, although still a symbol of medical authority, are now less commonly worn. Even in general practice the dress code is changing, with a general trend towards informality, and an increasing proportion of male general practitioners no longer wearing jacket and tie for consultations or home visits.

All of these changes diminish the distinction between doctor and patient and contribute towards demystification.

1.7.5.2 Varying styles of consultation

Many doctors have become less formal during the consultation. 'Doctors orders' is a phrase which entered common parlance but whose significance is now reduced, as doctors less commonly give strict 'orders'. Furthermore, clinicians now develop their own consulting styles, with training in general practice encouraging a participative style of shared decision-making.

A study of consulting style in the United States found that patients had different expectations which, unfortunately, were rarely matched by the clinician, with the implication being that each clinician develops his or her own consulting style and delivers it to all patients, whatever the individual patient's preferences may be. This issue will be discussed in more detail but its importance in the current context is that the general trend has been towards informality and openness with the physician trying to demystify the process of decision-making.

1.7.5.3 The mode of address

The patient who has known a doctor personally before the initial consultation, or before joining their list, will continue to use the doctor's first name, but the use of first names by both doctors and patients is increasing and doctors who look after patients on a long-term basis may develop a personal relationship, with the use of first names by both parties. Doctors are now more cautious about calling patients by their first name and less cautious about requesting patients to call them by their first name. This also contributes to demystification.

1.7.6 New healers are emerging

As doctors have become demystified, and have demystified themselves, other healers have emerged to fill the need for healing, and some of the criticism made of modern medicine derives from the fact that a patient may be looking both for the best of modern science and a traditional healer. As doctors in particular have become more like engineers, the patient's need for healing has not been met, causing dissatisfaction with the process of care (even though the patient is receiving the best technical quality), leaving the patient to seek other sources of healing as alternatives to the medical profession.

1.7.7 The charisma of the vulnerable human

The charisma of the remotely impressive doctor of the 20th century was powerful and had some beneficial effects for some patients, but for many the effect was demeaning. The charisma of that type of doctor derived from the reverence in which the profession was held, often augmented by the behaviour of the individual doctor. The diminution of this type of charisma may have been replaced by another type of charisma.

The word 'charisma' is now used to describe the superficial image of a public figure, closer to the adjective 'glamorous' than to the original meaning which referred to certain personal characteristics of the individual. The 21st century clinician, stripped back of the image from which 20th century charisma derived, can offer a substitute – his or her own, honest person, frailties and all. The doctor as superman has been replaced by the doctor as human being, willing to relate to another person – the patient – and the charisma of the human being who is the clinician may be as powerful as charisma derived from the false image.

Reference

(1) Lipkin, M. (1996) Sisyphus or Pegasus. *Ann. Intern. Med.*, 124: 511-13

Section 2

What do Doctors do all day?

Much attention has been given in the last decade to providing patients with more information about their health problems – about, for example, cancer, or depression, or psoriasis. This is obviously essential, but in addition to helping people understand disease we also need to help them understand clinical practice – how doctors think and make decisions, and how they interact with patients. Interaction is of particular importance because doctors interact with patients in a way that mechanics do not interact with machines, and this has an influence not only on the patient but also on the clinician.

Understanding disease and concepts such as cancer or atherosclerosis is obviously of great importance in improving communication, but nouns like 'cancer' and 'atherosclerosis' derived from the vast terminology of medicine have little connection with the consultation and the interaction between clinician and patient. The issue about how clinicians diagnose cancer or more subtle health problems like depression requires an understanding of the clinical process, what we may refer to as the grammar of medicine, as opposed to the vocabulary. In this section of the book the grammar of clinical practice is set out and the description of what doctors do all day gives an outline of what is happening in every consultation and every clinical decision. The various dimensions of what doctors do each day is described by analysing the clinical task in the way set out below.

2.1 'Let's open this chest fast'
2.2 The doctor as watchmaker – making a diagnosis
2.3 The doctor as watchmaker – appraising options
2.4 The doctor as tailor – applying research to the individual
2.5 The doctor as adviser – communicating information without framing
2.6 The doctor as witchdoctor – allaying anxiety
2.7 The doctor as St Peter – approving access to illness
2.8 The doctor as drug
2.9 The clinician as healer

2.1 'Let's open this chest fast'

The television programme *ER*, surely a major definer of the image of medicine in the year 2001, portrays the doctor's life as one of action. However, even surgeons, who epitomise action, rarely spend more than a quarter of their time actually in the operating theatre.

Research, education and, increasingly, management reduce the time the clinician spends in direct patient care. Even within the time identified as being preserved for clinical work, the act of treatment, either initiating it, operating, or providing long-term support to a patient with a chronic disease, occupies only part of the time spent on clinical duties – for many clinicians a minority of their time. A much larger proportion of time is spent on the steps leading up to treatment, namely:

- making a diagnosis;

- appraising the option of 'no treatment';

- comparing treatment options;

- tailoring the information to the individual patient;

- communicating information without framing;

- decision-making;

- decision-taking.

Furthermore, all these activities involve not only thinking but also feeling, and for many clinicians the steps leading up to treatment can be at least as difficult and stressful as carrying out the treatment itself. In some ways the need to act without thought when a patient arrives in ER bleeding profusely is, although stressful, less problematic for the doctor than acting as decision-maker when time pressures are not so great.

The best account currently available of what doctors do all day is provided by Jerome Groopman in his book *Second Opinions*. His book is a moving account of a number of cases, including that of his own child, illustrating how agonising and difficult clinical practice can be.

2.1.1 Overt and covert operations

The doctor carrying out the clinical duties described above is acting like a watchmaker, looking at the mind or body problem brought by the patient and seeking a solution to that problem. The watchmaker analogy only goes so far:

- because the human being is more complex to deal with than the watch: watches do not have anxieties and cannot sue;

- because the doctor's function of watchmaking is only their overt function.

The doctor also performs three covert functions while they are watchmaking and these may not be recognised either by the patient or the doctor even though they are important drivers of the consultation and clinical practice. These three covert functions are:

- the doctor as a witch doctor;

- the doctor as St Peter;

- the doctor as a drug.

Furthermore, the doctor, like other clinicians, has an additional function – that of healer. However, the principal reason why patients consult doctors is for the doctor to act as watchmaker.

2.2 The doctor as watchmaker – making a diagnosis

The clinician makes a diagnosis from data provided by:

- the patient's account of his symptoms;

- signs of disease observed by the patient or clinician;

- tests which produce numbers;

- tests which produce images.

The process is, however, more complicated than hunt-the-thimble because not all diseases are as clearly defined as a thimble, and there are numerous factors that the clinician has to bear in mind when making a diagnosis.

2.2.1 Two types of disease

Diseases are names given to conditions of the mind or body which medical experts agree to label as a disease, which are then included within the glossaries of diseases that they produce, for example the

Medical Subject Headings of the National Library of Medicine. However, experts may not agree on whether or not a condition is a disease.

Some diseases are unequivocally different from the normal condition, for example, fractured femur, tuberculosis and lung cancer. In other instances, people who are said to have a 'disease' simply have an exaggerated version of the normal condition, for example:

- if we say that someone has 'high blood pressure' it implies that they are qualitatively different from the general population, but

- everyone has a blood pressure, just as everyone has a height; however,

- some people's blood pressure is higher than others and

- in a proportion of the population, the level of blood pressure is sufficiently high to justify the person being offered treatment to reduce it, thus lessening the risk of stroke; such a person is said to 'have high blood pressure'.

Both types of disease have to be diagnosed using symptoms, signs or tests, and the accuracy of a symptom, sign or test is measured by its sensitivity and specificity.

2.2.2 The clinician must balance <u>sensitivity and specificity</u> when choosing a test

The two key characteristics of a test are sensitivity and specificity.

The sensitivity of a symptom, sign, or test is measured by the proportion of people who have the disease, among whom the test is positive.

The specificity is measured by the proportion of people without the disease, among whom the test is negative.

The ideal test should be 100% sensitive and 100% specific, but none are. Because of this, tests have false positives and false negatives.

However, the sensitivity and specificity of a test do not entirely define its usefulness. It is also important to assess the predictive value of a test.

2.2.3 When interpreting a test result, the <u>predictive values</u> of a test vary between hospital and general practice

The predictive value of a test is determined in part by its sensitivity, and in part by the prevalence of the disease in the population.

- The positive predictive value of a test is measured by the probability that someone with a positive test has the disease.

- The negative predictive value of a test is measured by the probability that someone with a negative test does not have the disease.

In general practice, for example, where many diseases are relatively uncommon, tests with a low sensitivity are often negative. Among patients referred to hospital, however, the predictive value of the test is much higher, because it is measured against a different group of people. This can lead to conflict between clinicians in primary and secondary care. In Jerome Groopman's account in *Second Opinions* of 'A Routine Case of Asthma', he recounts how he has to feed back to the primary care physician the fact that a diagnosis of leukaemia had been overlooked because the primary care physician had not confirmed the diagnosis of bronchitis, based on the patient's symptoms, with a laboratory test or a chest x-ray. As Dr Groopman said,

> 'We usually do that when symptoms don't respond to empiric therapy.'

> 'Dr Groopman, come down from your ivory tower and try working here in the trenches.' His voice spat acid and he recoiled in stunned silence. Rarely do physicians confront each other so directly.

> 'How many patients do you see in a week – six or maybe seven? – with residents and Fellows to do your scut work. Spend a week here with me; I have ten Isabella Monteras a day in the waiting room complaining in broken English that they need time off work because they are tired or can't breathe.'

> 'We have proven guidelines for what tests to order and what treatment to give. It is not cost-effective to do more than I did for a routine case of asthma. She wasn't bringing up sputum, her chest x-ray and blood count are outside our clinical algorithm for these cases. How many turn out to be a rare manifestation of leukaemia and leukostasis? For every thousand it's asthma in 999 plus times, so don't interrogate me.'

Differences in predictive value between hospital and primary care populations lead to:

- hospital clinicians accusing primary care clinicians of under-diagnosis, and

- primary care clinicians accusing hospital physicians of over-investigation.

Within both primary and secondary care there is a significant problem when diagnosis is based on human observation because observers vary in their detection rate of significant signs.

2.2.4 Inter-observer variability

Some images obviously indicate disease while others indicate absence of disease, but the problem in medicine often lies in grey zones and there are many images, for example x-rays or a pathology specimen, in which a number of different clinicians classify the same image differently. To some the image has a positive appearance whereas others classify it as a negative result. As a result, measurements of inter-observer variability are increasingly included in healthcare evaluation.

2.2.5 MUPS (medically unexplained physical symptoms)

Notwithstanding the weaknesses of diagnostic tests (which have only recently been recognised, but have always existed), it is now possible to diagnose accurately a much higher proportion of disease than in the past because of the power of modern diagnostic tools such as Magnetic Resonance Imaging (MRI). Many patients are therefore often reassured when no diagnosis is made. However, some patients are not reassured, and it is now understood that their symptoms can arise from a condition called MUPS, (medically unexplained physical symptoms), a recently recognised disorder, that also needs to be actively managed.

2.2.6 Bringing pathology face to face with patients

Clinical decisions can be classified as those which are made during the consultation – face to face decisions – and those which, at present, are made by a clinician remote from the patient. These latter, faceless, decisions are usually made by radiologists or pathologists who look at the image of a part of the patient – for example, a chest x-ray or a mammogram in the case of radiologists, or a cervical smear or lymph node removed during an operation in the case of pathologists. Alternatively, the decision about the patient may be made on the basis of some numbers calculated from the analysis of a patient's blood sample. This is what happens when a clinician sends a blood sample to the bio-chemistry laboratory. Haematologists making decisions about blood disease may make their faceless decisions on the basis of either an image, for example a slide on which the patient's blood cells can be examined under the microscope, or on the basis of numbers.

The reports produced by pathologists would be meaningless to most patients. There is, however, a movement among clinicians who are having to interpret the reports of pathologists and radiologists to force them to make their reports more comprehensible for both clinicians and patients. The clinicians who have to interpret these reports have pointed out the peculiar language used by pathologists, for example in a letter to *The Lancet* that was at the one time both humorous and serious, Dr Kay pointed out the incomprehensibility of systems for describing a certain type of lymphoma. [1]

> *Sir – The announcement in 'The Lancet' of two more classifications of non-Hodgkin's lymphomas encourages me to put forward my classification of these classifications.*
>
> *Well-defined, high grade, oligosyllabic.*
>
> *Poorly differentiated,*
>
> *polysyllabic –* $\begin{cases} \textit{diffuse} \\ \textit{circumlocutory} \\ \textit{with dyslexogenesis} \end{cases}$
>
> *Unicentric –* $\begin{cases} \textit{diffuse} \\ \textit{neologistic} \end{cases}$
>
> *Multicentric, cycnophilic*
>
> *Cleaved and convoluted types* ———$\begin{vmatrix} \textit{Rappaport} \\ \textit{(non-Lukes)} \\ \\ \textit{Lukes} \\ \textit{(non-Rappaport)} \end{vmatrix}$
>
> *This system makes no claim to be comprehensive or even comprehensible, so there may well be scope for other classifications of classifications and ultimately, one hopes, a classification of classifications of classifications. At that point we shall need a conference in the Caribbean.*
>
> *Yours sincerely,*
>
> *(Dr) H.E.M. Kay*

One solution to this has been to encourage those who make faceless decisions to be more straightforward in their systems of classification and the reports they write for clinical colleagues.

A second, more radical and more sensible, approach has been to suggest that pathologists start thinking about writing reports for patients. In a powerful editorial in *The Lancet*, one distinguished clinician suggested that pathologists had 'run amok' in describing carcinoma in situ of the breast. Elliott Foucar, an American pathologist, pointed out that the term 'carcinoma in situ' is often assumed by the patient to mean carcinoma, whereas it is more appropriate to consider the changes as representing a degree of risk rather than a clinical disease state. [2] His conclusion was that although pathology can be very difficult, 'it does not require specialised training in pathology to recognise that the patient's diagnosis should not be an anachronism sustained by anecdotes, conjecture, and tradition'. He called for a more honest description of the pathologist's observations and it would obviously be sensible to try to write these pathology reports both for the patient and for the clinician.

In biochemistry numbers are given out and expressed as lying within or outside a 'normal range'. The normal range, however, for a chemical in the bloodstream which has defined upper and lower limits is simply a description of the frequency of results. If, for example, the normal range is from 50 to 60, the person whose blood result is below 50 or above 60 may indeed have a disease but cannot be assumed to have a disease solely on the basis of their blood result, any more than the man who is below 5ft 5in or above 6ft 5in can be assumed to have a disease although they lie outside what could be called the normal range of height.

What is needed is for pathologists to summarise their findings so that they can be understood by patients. Admittedly that is a daunting task when one considers the wide range of educational levels of patients, but even if pathologists were to write their reports for no more than the 10 or 20 percent of patients who had a high school or university education, the discipline of doing so would not only force them to think of the consequences of the decision and bring them, if not face to face with the patient, at least directly in contact with the patient and the decision. Furthermore, from the complaints of clinicians about pathology results, if results were written to be comprehensible to the 10 or 20 percent of patients with high school or university education, they would almost certainly be more comprehensible for the general practitioners, physicians and surgeons who all too often find pathology reports difficult to interpret.

2.2.7 From diagnosis to action

Having made a diagnosis, the clinician has next to appraise options for action.

2.3 The doctor as watchmaker – appraising options

> *'I trust my lawyer more than my doctor; at least my lawyer sets out all the facts to me.'*
>
> *An American Patient*

> *Dr M diagnosed his own acoustic neuroma. He looked this up in the textbooks and accepted their advice that referral to an expert surgeon was necessary. He arranged an appointment and when he saw the surgeon, the surgeon told him that there was no-one more experienced in operating on the disease than himself. The operation was a success, so far as the removal of the tumour was concerned, but it permanently damaged the facial nerve.*

> *Years later Dr M discovered that 50% of acoustic neuromas do not grow quickly and that they can be safely monitored for a year or two after diagnosis to check the rate of growth. Thus an alternative to surgery would have been active surveillance with an annual MRI examination. Unfortunately the surgeon, although an expert at action, was poorly informed of work on the natural history of the disease and the option of not intervening was not considered.*
>
> *A British doctor's tale*

The doctor as watchmaker who has made a diagnosis has three questions to answer.

2.3.1 Active surveillance or active intervention?

Having made a diagnosis, there is often pressure to act. This is not always in the best interests of the patient, and the desire to act sometimes results not simply from a desire to please but from inadequate understanding of the natural history or prognosis of the untreated disease. This has led to a new slogan developing in medicine – *'Don't just do something, stand there'* as an antidote to decades, and perhaps centuries, of well-intentioned intervention without adequate understanding of natural history.

However, when intervention is necessary, the clinician has to appraise different options.

2.3.2 Option A or Option B?

Having decided that the condition should not be left untreated, the best treatment option has to be identified, and to do this the clinician has to:

- find all the relevant evidence by searching <u>Medline</u> or by using purified distillates of knowledge such as <u>The Cochrane Library</u>;
- appraise the evidence found, using <u>standardised checklists</u>.

2.3.3 Am I asking the right questions?

All this sounds very neat and logical but the treatment does not necessarily follow the diagnosis as night follows day because each patient is unique and may present a combination of risk factors and disease complications not covered by the research literature. Furthermore, in very rare diseases there may be no standardised treatment that can be followed or modified, as <u>Jerome Groopman</u> outlines in *Second Opinions* in his story called 'Don't just do something, stand there' in which he describes an argument between himself and another highly esteemed physician, one of whom believes the patient should have a transplant, the other wanting to try to stimulate the bone marrow. The language is often strong and direct, as, for example, when one expert says to the other, 'It's madness just to sit and wait for the next catastrophe.'

2.3.4 Tailoring research evidence

Evidence is derived from research, almost always based on the study of groups of patients. When the watchmaker is handed an Omega Seamaster he knows it will be identical to all other Seamasters. However, when the clinician sees a patient with stomach cancer or migraine, he can be equally sure that the patient in the consulting room will differ in many important ways from the patients in the research on stomach cancer or migraine. The clinician has to tailor the information to ensure that it will fit the needs of the particular patient.

2.4 The doctor as tailor – applying research to the individual

Stuff: material for making garments. (1462)
Bespoke: arranged for. (1583)
To tailor: to fit or furnish a person with clothes. (1832)

Shorter Oxford English Dictionary

Research produces 'stuff', information, and the knowledge revolution that has taken place in the last decade has not only indicated how the stuff produced by research has many imperfections, but has also demonstrated that the quality of the stuff can be greatly improved, initially by creating systematic reviews, and then by editing and clarifying the text that is produced. Although the quality of the product that has been created is increasingly improved by the process of purification and distillation known as <u>systematic reviewing</u>, research still produces 'stuff' which is no more useful for helping an individual patient make a decision than a roll of cloth is to the person who wishes to dress smartly for an important function.

Just as the tailor has to turn the stuff into garments arranged specifically for the individual person, so the clinician has to arrange the knowledge produced by research, even when its quality has been established, into a form fit for decision-making. This task has become more challenging as the stuff of research has become more plentiful and of a higher quality.

2.4.1 Tailoring 19th century stuff

In the 19th century, research products were fairly simple, usually consisting of reports of single cases or of small numbers of cases. In those days the clinician could only consider the degree to which their patient corresponded to the cases about which they had been taught or about which they had read, and make decisions accordingly. Unfortunately we now know that this approach to research gives <u>highly biased</u> results or results which could have occurred by <u>chance</u>.

2.4.2 Tailoring 20th century stuff

In the 20th century, clinical research methods developed dramatically, particularly in the latter half of the century as statistics were increasingly used.

The development of statistics took place not in medicine but in other sciences, notably in mathematics, from which statistics became a healthy offshoot, with the work being led by people like <u>Ronald Fisher</u>, whose classic designs for agricultural experiments later provided the model for clinical experiments. After the Second World War, the <u>randomised controlled trial</u> became prominent as a means of assessing the effectiveness of a new treatment of tuberculosis with streptomycin. The most important conceptual leap that statisticians made was to indicate that research had to focus not merely on single patients or small numbers of patients but on populations, namely a group of patients with common characteristics. This required an increasingly precise definition of the populations being studied, for example, the 'participants' in a trial of treatment for chronic obstructive lung disease were 'men and women aged between 40 and 70 years with a mean forced expiratory volume in one second (FEV1) 50% of predicted normal'. Patients were excluded from this study for a number of reasons if, for example, 'they used betablockers'. Consider now the problem of the clinician and the patient if the patient is 39 years old, or 72, or has used betablockers once at some time in the past.

One of the jobs of the clinician, therefore, is to take the knowledge derived from studies of populations and turn it into figures which are relevant to the individual, and this is one of the core skills of evidence-based clinical practice.

2.4.3 Evidence-based clinical practice

Evidence-based medicine developed during the 1990s, and has been defined as:

> ...the conscientious, explicit, and judicious use of current best evidence in making decisions about the care of individual patients. The practice of evidence based medicine means integrating individual clinical expertise with the best available external clinical evidence from systematic research. By individual clinical expertise we mean the proficiency and judgement that individual clinicians acquire through clinical experience and clinical practice. (3)

Key steps in evidence-based medicine are:

- asking the right question;
- finding the evidence;

- appraising the evidence;

- tailoring that evidence to be relevant and applicable to the individual patient.

Research often produces results stated as probabilities, indicating the relative benefit likely to be achieved from the treatment. There is, however, good evidence that providing information about the relative reduction of risk biases decision-making, a phenomenon called framing, and it is therefore essential to turn the information into absolute figures; this is one of the jobs of the clinician as tailor.

2.4.4 Giving patients information about absolute risk reduction

The first step the clinician as tailor has to take is to turn relative risk data into absolute risk data, and the technique used to do this is called the number needed to treat (NNT). This indicates the number of patients who have to be treated for one patient to benefit, and the technique has been well described and popularised by the journal *Bandolier*. Even having converted the data into absolute figures, the clinician still has to tailor it to the individual patient and the book *Evidence-based Medicine* gives guidance as to how important results from a research perspective might be applicable to a particular patient (Table 1).

Table 1: Are these valid, important results applicable to our patient?

Is our patient so different from those in the study that its results cannot apply?

Is the treatment feasible in our setting?

What are our patient's potential benefits and harms from the therapy?

What are our patient's values and expectations for both the outcome we are trying to prevent and the treatment we are offering?

Sackett et al, Evidence-Based Medicine [4]

The clinician then has to follow the same process of:

- producing data about the absolute risk of harm, if only the relative risks are given in the scientific paper, and;

- considering the applicability of the <u>number to needed to harm</u> (<u>NNH</u>), namely the number who were treated for one to be harmed, and then seeking to assess the relevance of those data to the individual patient, using a checklist such as that set out below (Table 2).

Table 2: Guides for deciding whether valid important evidence about harm can be applied to our patient

Is our patient so different from those in the study that its results don't apply?

What is our patient's risk of the adverse event? What is our patient's potential benefit from the therapy?

What are our patient's preferences, concerns and expectations from this treatment?

What alternative treatments are available?

Sackett et al, Evidence-Based Medicine [2]

2.4.5 Integrating preferences and values

Having provided the patient with the best data available, tailored to his or her particular condition, the clinician then has to help the patient weigh up the options and decide the value that they will assign to either a beneficial or an adverse outcome. An example of this approach in practice is given in the resources section describing the tailoring of information about aspirin, where the data apparently indicate a simple decision but in which the patient's condition, which determines the relevance of the data to him as an individual, and his values and preferences, have to be incorporated.

Because of the complexity of the process, different approaches have been used to develop decision aids to facilitate some of these steps.

2.4.6 The legal view of risk communication

The degree to which the doctor should disclose risk is also influenced by the courts because doctors and their employers are mindful of the possible legal consequences of any failure to disclose risk. For years legal judgements on negligence have been made with respect to the Bolam principle which was established in a case in 1957 and which states that medical actions and decisions are justifiable if they are 'in accordance with a practice accepted by a responsible body of medical men.' However, the courts are not bound by this principle, recognising that such a consensus may not be based on best current evidence, and a judgement by Lord Woolf provides the principle on which courts will accept the adequacy of the consent procedure.

The judgement, in the Pearce case in 1999, states that: 'If there is a significant risk which would affect the judgement of a reasonable patient then … it is the responsibility of a doctor to inform the patient of that risk if the information is needed so that the patient can determine … what course he or she should adopt.' By 'significant', the defence societies advise that the doctor should consider risks with a frequency of 1% or greater, and all risks of death or serious complications, no matter how rarely they occur. Lord Woolf's Pearce judgement also states that the clinician needs to ask himself or herself: 'Is there a significant risk which would affect the judgement of a reasonable patient in this situation, which has not been disclosed, and which I need to convey to my patient so that he or she can determine what course to adopt?'

In Australia, clearer guidance has been given, summarised in the box below.

Relevant factors
(The high court of Australia considers the following factors important in deciding whether a risk is material and must be mentioned to a patient.
(*The nature of the matter to be disclosed* – More likely and more serious harms require disclosure.
(*The nature of the proposed procedure* – Complex interventions require more information, as do procedures where the patient has no illness.
(*The patient's desire for information* – Patients who ask questions make known their desire for information and should be told.
(*The temperament and health of the patient* – Anxious patients and patients with health problems or other relevant circumstances that make a risk more important for them (such as their medical condition or occupation) may need more information.
(*The general surrounding circumstances* – The information necessary for elective procedures, where several consultations are possible, may be different from that required in an emergency department.

Recognising that the recollection of what patient and clinician said, never mind what they understood, during the consultation, which may have taken place months or years before the complaint or the court case, clinicians are also exhorted to keep good records of the consultation, but paper has its limitations and for difficult decisions a tape recording may provide the best record, as recommended in the enquiry into the cardiac surgery deaths in Bristol.

2.5 The doctor as adviser – communicating information without framing

Frame: To fake the result of a race etc. (1910)

Shorter Oxford English Dictionary

People are framed by circumstantial evidence but data can be framed as well, and the framing of data can influence decision-making, particularly when it is so easy, using modern statistical software, to change the way in which data is presented. Furthermore, it is extremely easy, using the Web, for pharmaceutical companies to present data to clinicians and patients in ways most likely to influence the decision to prescribe; of central importance in successful framing is the use of relative rather than absolute risk reduction data.

2.5.1 Distinguishing between absolute and relative risk reduction

People who particularly wish to influence others, as opposed to letting them make up their own minds, often choose to express the data as what is called a relative risk reduction.

For example, in the late eighties, following the publication of a meticulously organised randomised controlled trial of the effects of lipid-lowering drugs on mortality from coronary heart disease, an advertisement claimed that the drug 'reduces coronary heart disease risk by 34%.' At about the same time, another study carried out in Helsinki was published, and the two articles together led to what was called 'an unprecedented wave of enthusiasm for treating patients who have hypercholesterolaemia', raised levels of cholesterol in the bloodstream.

However, the results of the research were able to be presented in two ways, as shown in Table 3.

Table 3: Ways of presenting research for hypercholesterolaemia				
	1	2	3	4
	% having heart attacks in the group which did not receive lipid lowering drugs (the control group)	% having heart attacks in the group which did receive lipid lowering drugs (the intervention group)	Absolute risk reduction (2-3)	Relative risk reduction ARR x 100 % in the control group
Lipid Research Centres Trial	9.8%	8.1%	1.7%	19%
Helsinki Trial	4.1%	2.7%	1.4%	34%

Brett, A.S. 'Treating hypercholesterolemia' [5]

Column 1 shows the rate of heart attacks in the control group which did not receive the lipid lowering drugs, and column 2 the rate in the group which did receive the lipid lowering drugs.

Column 3 is the absolute reduction in risk which is the difference in the percentages of patients having heart attacks in the two groups.

The relative risk reduction (Column 4) takes the absolute risk reduction and converts it into a percentage of the percentage of patients having heart attacks in the group not receiving the lipid lowering drugs, called the control group by research workers.

The presentation of research results as either absolute or relative risk reduction has dramatic effects on decision-making by patients, clinicians and policy makers.

2.5.2 The impact of relative risk reduction on patient decision-making

One hundred Torontonian outpatients were asked whether or not they would take lipid lowering drugs. They were offered 'information' in two different ways – as either relative, or absolute, risk reduction. The difference in the responses of the two groups is striking, as shown in Table 4, and other studies have shown the same effect. [6,7]

Table 4	
Methods of expressing the reduction in risk	**Percentage of patients choosing treatment**
'34% Reduction in heart attacks' (Relative risk reduction)	88%
'1.4% reduction in heart attacks' (Absolute risk reduction)	42%

Hux, J.E. and Naylor, C.D.[8]

In one study, [9] 56.8% of patients chose medication when the benefit was expressed in relative terms, more than three times the 14.7% who chose the medication when the benefit was expressed in absolute terms.

2.5.3 Physicians and policy-makers can be misled by framing

2.5.3.1 Misleading physicians

Physicians too are influenced by framing and three studies [7,10,11] all demonstrated that physicians were more influenced by relative than by absolute risk reduction.

2.5.3.2 Misleading the experts

Few clinicians have received extensive training in epidemiology; their concern is for individuals rather than populations. However, even decision-makers whose job is to appraise decisions from the perspective of the population rather than the individual, are influenced by framing. A research team presented 182 health authority members with the results from randomised trials on breast cancer screening and a systematic review of trials of cardiac rehabilitation. They presented the results in four different ways, as shown in Table 5.

Table 5: Testing the framing effect – presentation of the same information about two programmes in four different ways

Information presentation	Mammography	Cardiac rehabilitation
Relative risk reduction	34%	20%
Absolute risk reduction	0.06%	3%
Percentage of event-free patients	99.82% vs 99.8%	84% vs 87%
Number needed to treat (NNT)	1592	31

Fahey et al, Evidence-based purchasing[12]

140 of the 182 decision-makers returned questionnaires and demonstrated clearly that their willingness to fund both programmes was influenced significantly by the way in which the results were presented; again they opted for relative risk reduction. Especially worryingly, perhaps, for the trained epidemiologists, in the group being studied, only 3 of the 140 'all non-executive members claiming no training in epidemiology' spotted that the four sets of data expressed the same results in different ways.

2.5.4 Giving information in words, numbers, images and hieroglyphs

Recognising that words can often be interpreted in different ways, particularly adverbs of probability such as 'probably' and 'possibly', numbers are increasingly used to influence decisions. It has long been recognised that basic numeracy skills vary in the population and those who are less numerate, not surprisingly, have more difficulty in appreciating options. [13] However, numeracy alone is not enough; clinicians, patients and all decision-makers in health and healthcare need to understand the impact of framing, particularly when clinicians are committed to shared decision-making.

2.5.5 Promoting the understanding of absolute risk reduction

Fortunately the concepts of absolute and relative risk reduction are easy to understand and the importance of presenting information to clinicians, patients and policy makers is now accepted and is being promoted.

The absolute benefits of treatments can be described in terms of the Number Needed to Treat (NNT) and examples of this are shown in Table 6.

Table 6: NNTs for various interventions
Source: extracts from Bandolier 1995; 17:7, and McQuay and Moore[12]

Intervention	Outcome	NNT
CABG in left main stenosis	Prevent 1 death at 2 years	6
Carotid endarterectomy in high grade symptomatic stenosis	Prevent 1 stroke or death in 2 years	9
Simple antihypertensive therapy for severe hypertension	Prevent 1 stroke, MI or death in 1 year	15
Simple antihypertensive therapy for mild hypertension	Prevent 1 stroke, MI or death in 1 year	700
Treating hypertension in the over-60s	Prevent 1 coronary event	18
Aspirin in severe unstable angina	Prevent MI or death in 1 year	25
Aspirin in healthy US physician	Prevent MI or death in 1 year	500
Graduated compression stockings for venous thromboembolism	Episodes of venous thrombo-embolism	9
Triple therapy for peptic ulcer	Eradication of H. pylori	1.1
Triple therapy for peptic ulcer	Ulcers remaining cured at 1 year	1.8
Permethrin for headlice	Cure	1.1
Antibiotics for dogbite	Infection	16

In the United Kingdom, increased professional awareness of the NNT is principally due to the excellent and highly readable journal *Bandolier,* and a visit to its website allows the reader to find many examples of the number needed to treat and its converse, the NNH – the number needed to harm.

The concept of absolute benefit is also being given prominence, for example when clinicians who feel that the public are being misled by newspaper headlines take the trouble to write to the press. An example of this was the excellent letter published in the *Glasgow Herald* which had headlined the relative risk reduction claims of a group of research workers:

> *Your report (August 16) on the trial published in this week's New England Journal of Medicine correctly states that in combination treatment with aspirin and clopido-grel in a selected group of high-risk patients, the relative reduction in risk of death, heart attack, and stroke was 20%. It is important to note that these events happened to 11.4% of patients receiving aspirin alone compared to 9.3% of patients receiving the two drugs together; an absolute reduction of 2.1%.*
>
> *You quote one of the researchers saying that this treatment is simple and safe. Simple perhaps but examination of the trial shows that major bleeding occurred in 2.7% of those receiving aspirin alone and 3.7% of those receiving aspirin plus clopi-dogrel. This was an absolute increase in risk of 1% and a relative increase in risk of 38%.*
>
> *Major bleeding was defined as substantially disabling, intraocular bleeding leading to loss of vision or bleeding necessitating the transfusion of at least two units of blood.*
>
> *Please note the editorial piece on the website –*
>
> *(http://content.nejm.org/this_week/345/7/index.shtml). 'Although clopidogril plus aspirin had clinical benefit beyond that of aspirin alone, the benefit was small and was partially offset by an increased risk of bleeding, including bleeding necessitating transfusion."*
>
> *Researchers are recommending doctors to start prescribing this immediately and not to wait for the combination to become licensed.*
>
> *But doctors are always legally responsible for the effects of drugs that they prescribe and if they prescribe a drug outwith its licence, their professional responsibility alters and increases. The Medical and Dental Defence Union of Scotland states: 'Although the Medicines Act allows doctors to recommend the use of drugs outside the param-eters of their licences, it does not mean that the doctor thus advised has to prescribe any drug recommended. If they feel that the use of any recommended drug is beyond their experience or knowledge they are under no obligation to prescribe it.*
>
> *Developments in the drug treatment of coronary events are welcomed, but the reporting of their benefits must be balanced with the clear safety issues.*
>
> Audrey Thompson, Medicines Management Adviser
> Dr Andrew Power, Head of Medicines Management,
> Gartnavel Royal Hospital, Glasgow.

Doctors sometimes consciously modify the information they give to patients with the best of intentions, and a study of the language used in the consultation demonstrated that doctors used phrases such as 'what they call' or adjectives such as 'little' to minimise the possible impact of terms such as fibro-adenoma and cervical erosion. The use of such terms is kindly meant but can sustain the imbalance of power between clinician and patient, maintaining the paternalistic power of the clinician and the childlike status of the patient, who responds by using phrases such as 'I was wondering' instead of asking direct questions.

2.5.6 The doctor as human being

The doctor here is portrayed as a logical calculating machine, relating to the patient as the watchmaker relates to the watch. The consultation, however, is different: it is an interaction between human beings, and the patient is influenced by the human elements of this interaction, partly because many patients bring more than one problem to the consultation – the sign or symptom that has led them to seek help as well as their anxiety about it.

2.6 The doctor as witchdoctor - allaying anxiety

Anxiety is a normal reaction to disease or the possibility of disease, and anxiety usually, but not always, leads the individual to seek professional help to resolve the uncertainty. If no disease is found, anxiety is usually, but not universally, allayed and the person continues with their life (Figure 8).

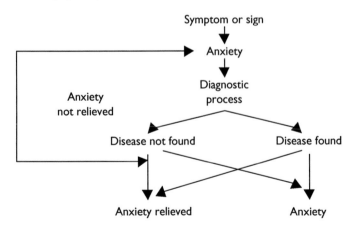

Figure 8

However, anxiety of different types can persist and aggravate the patient's problems.

2.6.1 Anxiety generated by disease

For some people the diagnosis of a disease comes as a relief. They feel empowered by the knowledge and look forward with confidence to treatment and cure. For others, even when an effective cure is available, diagnosis does not end anxiety, and the emotional response to illness is determined by a number of different factors such as:

- the severity of the disease;

- the effectiveness of available treatment;

- the side effects of available treatment;

- the confidence that the patient has in their clinician and health services;

- the patient's personality – some people are more disposed to anxiety than others.

When anxiety persists it can aggravate the symptoms of disease (Figure 9).

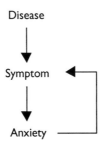

Figure 9

2.6.2 Medically unexplained physical symptoms can cause, and be aggravated by, anxiety

When no diagnosis is made – that is, no disease is found, because failure to diagnose is no guarantee of absence of disease – most people are relieved, but for a proportion of people anxiety persists, and can maintain or even increase the severity of the symptom (Figure 10).

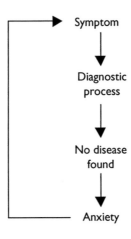

Figure 10

The probability of this happening is determined by a number of factors including:

- fear of a particular disease, fear of cancer being a major cause of anxiety;

- the personality of the individual;

- the way in which the symptoms, the diagnostic process, and the giving of information, have been managed.

2.6.3 Anxiety alone may be the cause of the patient's symptom

Some symptoms are actually caused by anxiety, and if the symptom which led the individual to consult the clinician in the first place was the result of anxiety, then failure to resolve their anxiety will tend to aggravate the symptom. Furthermore, anxiety itself can produce physical changes in the body. Psychosomatic diseases are those in which anxiety can actually cause a disease or, more commonly, aggravate the severity of the condition; asthma is an example of such a condition (Figure 11).

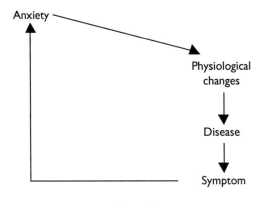

Figure 11

2.6.4 *The management of anxiety*

The management of anxiety, whether or not the diagnosis is known and whether or not the individual has a disease, is of central importance in healthcare and clinical practice. The best approach is, of course, to deal with all the underlying issues: accurate diagnosis, clear communication, and effective treatment, all carried out in a competent, caring way, are effective means of managing anxiety but it is also important to recognise that the organisation of healthcare and the style of the clinician can increase, as well as allay, anxiety. Anxiety arises from uncertainty, and modern medicine, although increasingly accurate in its diagnosis and more confident in the probability that treatment will be beneficial, is actually based on scientific methods in which the testing and refining of uncertainty are of central importance.

- Research produces conclusions which are statements of probability, not statements of certainty.

- What a modern clinician knows are not facts but probabilities.

The problems that uncertainty pose are vividly described in a doctor's account of his encounter with uncertainty:

We are encouraged these days to have more patient centred consultations, to share out thought processes and decision making with our patients, and to build therapeutic alliances. However, sharing uncertainty is not something I always find to be straightforward.

49

Six months ago, my perspective on uncertainty was radically changed and my ability to cope with it questioned like never before. I was diagnosed with non-Hodgkin's lymphoma. This was uncertainty of an entirely different order. This was me, for God's sake! I'm only 41. I've got a wife and children! This isn't how it was meant to be.

From the beginning, the rollercoaster of emotions that accompanies such a diagnosis and the progression through chemotherapy has been paralleled by the need to grapple with facts and figures. And how many times have I mulled over the discovery of that solitary cervical lymph node? It's probably nothing, I thought. Oh God, it's getting bigger – I need to do something. The histology shows low grade follicular lymphoma – good, that has longer survival rates. Bad – it's generally considered to be incurable. A scan reveals abdominal nodes. But wait – the bone marrow is clear! I pore over complex classifications of lymphomas and their seemingly endless revisions. I devour the recent publications on the treatment of follicular lymphomas. I scour the internet for that elusive article that will reveal all and restore hope. The doctor in me looks coldly at the statistics and is overcome with pessimism. What is the five year survival rate for a 41 year old man without lymphoma anyway? The patient in me prefers to look at the bottle and find it half full. There are a lot of promising developments in treatment, I tell myself.

Tom Cuddihy[14]

In shared decision-making, these probabilities or uncertainties are shared with the patient, but not all patients welcome that: some wish to have an authoritative figure, preferring the certainty that the traditional clinician exuded so well.

2.6.5 Clinical practice – science or magic?

Anthropologists have defined the function of magic as the management of anxiety when no effective intervention is available. Scientifically, it is known that rain dances do not bring rain, but the rain dance provided a useful, apparently purposeful, activity for the community waiting for rain. Rain, of course, ultimately falls, reinforcing belief in the rain dance and thus increasing its effectiveness as a means of relieving anxiety still further.

- The 19th century clinician relied principally on magic.

- The 20th century clinician used science consciously and magic unconsciously, although many clinicians were aware of the need to allay anxiety and used the power of the drug doctor frequently and with beneficence.

- The 21st century clinician is less willing to do so, and some regard the practice as unethical and paternalistic.

From the perspective of the patient, however, the need for magic may be greater than ever before.

2.6.6 The growing need for magic

If magic is a means of managing uncertainty, this need is determined in part by the amount of uncertainty in life in general – and life is becoming increasingly uncertain. As <u>Ulrich Beck</u> has described graphically, the world of work is changing, with decreasing job security, in what he calls the '<u>Brazilianisation of the West</u>'. Furthermore, he pointed out in his monumental work *The Risk Society* that everyone was at risk in an increasingly uncertain environment. Faced with increasing uncertainty, individuals need reassurance and support, and if they do not find it from a clinician perhaps understandably unwilling to act as a witch doctor, they may turn to alternative medicine.

2.6.7 Alternative medicine

The complementary or alternative sector of the healthcare industry is growing faster than any other. The definition of complementary and alternative, and even conventional or orthodox medicine, can be subdivided into four types of care:

- necessary;
- appropriate;
- inappropriate;
- futile.

2.6.7.1 Necessary care

Necessary care is that which is universally agreed as being necessary. Even <u>Ivan Illich</u>, who first articulated a criticism of mainstream medicine in his polemic *The Limits of Medicine* accepted the need for someone to deal with severe toothache or a broken leg. Necessary care is:

- defined by society as a high priority;
- recognised as a need by all doctors;

● funded in almost every developed country.

Pain control would be regarded as necessary care.

2.6.7.2 *Appropriate medical care*

After necessary care, it is possible to define appropriate care on the spectrum. This is care in which:

● there is a good probability of doing more good than harm;

● it is regarded as a reasonable standard of care in the context of the society.

Coronary artery bypass grafting and hip replacement, for example, are regarded as appropriate care in every developed country for people with, respectively, myocardial ischaemia or osteoarthrosis of the hip. Failure to provide such care would be seen as a serious dereliction of duty on the part of the individual clinician or the health service.

2.6.7.3 *Inappropriate care*

Inappropriate care is that deemed unreasonable in a particular context or for a particular individual.

For example, teflon fibre grafts to replace the cruciate ligaments of the knee are appropriate for a professional ice hockey player whose income and career depend upon a stable knee joint, but could be deemed inappropriate for the person who finds knee instability irksome and wishes to play tennis once every couple of months without the feeling that a knee will collapse.

It is important to distinguish between inappropriate care for the individual and an inappropriate use of finite resources.

In societies in which resources are finite, the definition of inappropriateness is made with respect to the opportunity costs of providing such services, namely what else could be done with the money. If, for example, there were a waiting list for coronary artery bypass grafting, it would not be appropriate to spend limited resources on an elaborate orthopaedic intervention to facilitate occasional mild physical exercise as a leisure pursuit.

For the individual, however, what is regarded as inappropriate by society as a whole may be highly desirable. This applies to aesthetic surgery, for example straightening or reducing the nose, or enlarging or reducing the breasts. If an individual is demonstrably severely depressed by some aspect of their appearance, perhaps suicidally so, then it may be appropriate to use finite resources to help that individual, but if the main wish of the individual is to increase their sexual attractiveness, many people would regard that as being an inappropriate use of resources.

2.6.7.4 Futile care

At the other end of the spectrum from necessary care is futile care, which:

- does not accord with the patient's wishes, and

- would be regarded as inappropriate by most clinicians.

Radical surgery, intended to be curative but with no evidence of benefit, for a patient with advanced cancer who has requested control of symptoms, is an example of futile care.

2.6.7.5 Complementary medicine

There is no universally agreed definition of complementary medicine but one definition is that it consists of care of which many - perhaps most - physicians approve, and to which they would refer patients, but which is not automatically paid for by the state or insurance companies.

Examples of complementary medicine include:

- homeopathy;

- osteopathy;

- chiropractic.

Aesthetic surgery, which people can now access online, could, of course, also be added to this list and the definition is determined to a degree by the extent of state funding. For example, thirty years ago the National Health Service provided basic foot care to all older people free of charge. However, as the population has aged, services have not expanded and older people now only receive podiatry if they have some particular condition, for example, diabetes or vascular disease. Those who are unable to give themselves basic foot care, for example because of osteoarthritis of the hips, are required to pay for it or are referred to private chiropodists by primary care professionals. Thus basic foot care can now be regarded as a form of complementary medicine.

2.6.7.6 *Alternative medicine*

Alternative implies that individuals should choose either standard healthcare, with or without complementary medicine, or the alternative. There is, however, evidence that patients use both simultaneously. Increasingly the distinction between complementary and alternative medicine is blurring and one proposal is to consider the two as a single entity of Complementary and Alternative Medicine (CAM). [15]

A pragmatic definition of alternative medicine is that it is a form of care, usually based on an alternative biological paradigm, which some physicians actively encourage, whereas an increasing number of others are sympathetic towards it as long as it does not lead the patient to refuse conventional treatment for a disorder for which conventional treatment exists. Acupuncture, Chinese medicine, and vitamin therapy are examples of alternative medicine.

In addition to these generic types of alternative medicine there are a multitude of specific systems, sometimes linked to one individual, such as, for example:

- Dr Andrew Weil's methods;

- Dr Gerson's cancer therapy.

2.6.7.7 *People use alternative medicine for different reasons*

The fact that people use both mainstream medicine and alternative medicine indicates that at least some of the people who use alternative medicine do so not simply because they have become dissatisfied with conventional health care, but because they find additional value in the alternative approach.

Four types of reason are given by those who use alternative health care.

- **Certainty.** Part of the approach of empowering patients in mainstream medicine is to involve them in shared decision-making. In explaining options fully, uncertainty is usually clearly described, namely the fact that there is a probability of benefit and a probability of harm and (if more detail is asked for) that the evidence on which these probabilities are calculated is itself derived from research which can only produce an estimate of the extent of the good or bad effect. Alternative medicine is usually less uncertain medicine and for those who wish certainty, alternative medicine is a better option.

- *Personalisation.* Mainstream medicine uses knowledge derived from the studies of groups, and decisions are made on the basis that, for example, aspirin has been shown to reduce mortality among people with cerebrovascular disease. Thus people with cerebrovascular disease should be considered for aspirin treatment. The patient is compared with the group and decisions are based on how other people with the same disease have been treated. Increasingly the weakness of this approach, applied uncritically, has been exposed, for example, by the evidence-based medicine movement. A closer examination of the benefits of aspirin illustrates the need to tailor knowledge to the individual patient.

In contrast, many forms of alternative medicine focus on the individual, not only in terms of the time and personal attention given to the patient but also in terms of basing decisions on the constitution of the individual, rather than the similarity of the patient to the group. Homeopathy, for example, is based on the principle that the constitutional type of the individual has to be established as a basis for all intervention.

- *Evidence.* There is evidence that alternative medicine is beneficial. Some people, particularly those with health problems that do not fit neatly into conventional systems of classification, report tremendous benefit. Their testimony encourages them to continue using alternative medicine, usually a particular type which they have found beneficial, and also encourages those to whom they describe their success to do so also.

Those in mainstream medicine usually attribute these successes either to the placebo effect or to the reduction in anxiety that certainty brings, or some combination of these factors, but for the individual the evidence of benefit is evidence enough.

- *Alternative 'Weltanschauungen'.* The 'Weltanschauung', or world view, of most people in mainstream medicine is firmly rooted in a certain view of reality, one that sees reality from the perspective of

- a reductionist approach to science;

- a split between mind and body;

- a dualism that also emphasises the distinction between self and other, between subjective and objective.

This is, however, only one way of looking at the world, and there are many others. A natural consequence of this approach has been the belief that science is good and progress is good, although this is now no longer held so simply as it was in the confident days of the early 1960s when it seemed that science could solve all problems. In the new world, most clearly described by the sociologist Ulrich Beck, science is seen as having adverse as well as beneficial effects and alternative world views are recognised as having their own validity. There is some evidence that some people choose alternative medicine because they prefer the world view, the Weltanschauung, offered by Buddhism or Taoism or by an individual clinician whom they regard, in the appropriate use of the word, as a guru.

2.6.7.8 Integrative medicine

Attitudes towards complementary and alternative medicine are changing within mainstream medical care and increasingly the value of these other approaches is being recognised not only by patients but also by clinicians.

One formulation developed by Dr Andrew Weil, alternative medicine's first superstar, who topped the *New York Times* best-seller list and appeared on the front cover of *Time* magazine, is that we should be using what he calls 'integrative medicine'. This is using mainstream medicine for what it is good at doing – such as fixing broken legs, bypassing narrow arteries and treating childhood leukaemia – while recognising that other approaches can help alleviate the suffering that many patients find not only unrelieved by conventional health care but also actually aggravated by the loss of power that they experience by becoming 'just a number' in a huge machine as awesome and impersonal as the *Metropolis* of Fritz Lang.

2.7 The doctor as St Peter – approving access to illness

The doctor has not only to act as watchmaker: often he is also a gatekeeper, guarding the entrance to specialist care or to the state of illness.

2.7.1 Having and being – disease and illness

A person has a disease but is ill: a disease is something you have, illness is an altered state of being.

Although the words 'disease' and 'illness' are sometimes used as synonyms, most people appreciate the distinction between them, even though they have never read the work of sociologists like <u>Talcott Parsons</u> and <u>David Mechanic,</u> who analysed and described the concept of illness and the behaviour associated with it.

2.7.2 Illness has privileges

Ill people have power and enjoy two types of privileges because of that power:

- increased sympathy and attention, and
- freedom from normal societal obligations such as working, or attending school.

2.7.3 Illness also has rules

The 'rewards' of illness are obviously attractive and it is not surprising that some people seek to become ill even though they have no disease. Society has a whole set of checks and balances to regulate illness behaviour as anyone who has been a parent well knows – for example: 'if you don't go to school on Friday, you cannot go out to the disco on Saturday'. Similar rules apply for adults: those who claim the benefits of illness have to display the following behaviours:

- trying to get better, that is conforming to lay or medical advice;
- relinquishing normal social pleasures such as going out to the cinema or parties;
- going to see the doctor if the state of illness lasts more than a few days.

Miss A was a schoolteacher who had frequent short-term sickness absences from the school in which she worked. She usually seemed in the best of health and these short-term absences were a considerable annoyance to her colleagues because they were rarely accompanied by a sick note from the doctor. However, for several years her behaviour had been tolerated without explicit comment from colleagues or the

Headmaster until the occasion when, after being off work ill on Thursday and Friday, she was photographed sitting proudly on the first ever Park and Ride bus to go into the city centre at 8.30 on the Saturday morning, smugly celebrating her small place in history, preserved in a photograph for the local paper. Her colleagues at school, however, found it completely unacceptable that someone who had been off sick on Thursday and Friday should have recovered so dramatically by the Saturday morning, and on her return to school on Monday morning she received both direct criticism from her colleagues and a disciplinary talk from her Headmaster.

To be recognised as really ill, the claimant has to have their claim validated by a doctor, and the 21st century doctor has many more powerful tools to confirm or refute the claim by diagnosing a disease that can explain the patient's symptoms and feelings of illness.

2.7.4 Going to see the doctor to validate real illness

The right to claim the privileges of illness is open to all, but only for a limited period of time. The individual who claims he or she is 'really ill' and unable to work, either for pay or within the household, will not be allowed to claim the privileges for long without being advised, encouraged or required to see the doctor by those who have to shoulder the consequences by doing extra work themselves.

This advice, encouragement, or requirement is sometimes made in the best interests of the person claiming the rights of illness, but it is not for nothing that the word 'pretender' came to mean more than its original definition of 'claimant' and is now imbued with the implication of acting. The person who pretends to be ill is required to undergo a test to make sure they are not acting, and the doctor carries out that test, rarely enthusiastically, because many doctors are annoyed that they have to operate the rule and act as lie detector, distinguishing those who are really ill from those who should be denied the rights of illness and returned to their normal societal obligations when a bid for the power that comes from being recognised as really ill is thwarted.

The doctor is expected to act like St Peter, holding the keys to illness, to unlock the door through which many wish to pass.

2.7.5 Doctors as society's risk managers

Doctors, general practitioners in particular, are sometimes described as gatekeepers, deciding which patients shall be referred to hospital. The term 'gatekeeper' implies that the job of the doctor is to separate those who need specialist care from those who do not, as the shepherd separates ewes from lambs when shedding his flock. The doctor's job is not, however, as easy as the shepherd's. It is sometimes easy to distinguish the patients who need specialist care but often it is not. The general practitioner who has some anxiety about the child who is ill or the patient who feels tired could make a referral, but they may desist to spare the patient unnecessary tests and anxiety, and to spare the hospital service from work with which it could not cope. The doctor, however, has to carry the anxiety that results from the decision not to refer. The anxiety may not be great for any single decision but the cumulative effect of the hundreds of decisions of this sort is a heavy burden that the doctor bears for society in managing these risks.

2.7.6 Being ill in the 21st century

More people can now validate illness. Because of the growing workload of doctors, their gatekeeper function is being reduced, and self-certification of illness is now an option for many employees. In addition, there are now numbers of other health professionals whose word will be taken as evidence of real illness, ranging from those whose credibility is almost universally accepted, such as the chiropractor or the homeopathic clinician, to those whose validation is not generally recognised, for example the acupuncturist or the herbalist whose opinions will be accepted by friends if not by the employer.

The increase in the power of medicine to diagnose disease is also changing the passage to illness in the 21st century, making it more difficult. Consider the person who tells his doctor that he has no energy and feels weak. These symptoms could be due to a wide range of different diseases – tuberculosis, cancer, or thyroid disease. In the 19th century, diagnostic accuracy was limited and the fact that the doctor could not diagnose a disease did not mean that no disease was present. In the last hundred years this has changed, and if the doctor uses the full range of diagnostic tests and finds no sign of disease, the probability that the person has a disease, although it exists, is very low. If the doctor can find nothing wrong, the symptoms may disappear, but they may persist in a condition called MUPS – medically unexplained physical symptoms – and the person may also find it very difficult to be accepted as being really ill unless he seeks another clinician to validate his claim, or enters the shadowy lands of illnoids – hypochondriasis and malingering.

2.7.7 Anxiety as illness, clinician as treatment

Because the patient's symptoms may stem solely from, or be aggravated by, anxiety, the interaction with the doctor can, if it alleviates anxiety, cure or mitigate the problem – with the doctor acting as the drug.

2.8 The doctor as drug

The Tavistock Clinic, a world famous centre for psychotherapy research and practice, now occupies an unprepossessing concrete building which sticks out like a sore thumb among the redbrick villas of Hampstead. In the 1950s, however, the Tavistock Clinic was based in Hallam Street, in the Tavistock Estate, that part of London south of the Euston Road and north of Oxford Street, including Bloomsbury and Fitzrovia, which was the heartland of the capital's intellectual life in the 20th century. One of the luminaries of the Tavistock Clinic, the psychotherapist Michael Balint, worked with a number of general practitioners in what became known as Balint groups, which destroyed for ever the concept of the doctor as watchmaker.

2.8.1 Patients consult doctors for many reasons

Patients consult doctors for many reasons but until the insights provided by the Balint groups, it was assumed that patients took their health problem along to the doctor in the same way as they took a watch along to the watchmaker when it no longer kept good time. The job of the doctor, like that of the watchmaker, was to identify the cause of the problem and fix it, returning health to the patient like the well functioning watch which was returned to the customer after it was repaired or cleaned. The Balint groups, however, started to articulate a new way of looking at consultations and gave a clear and explicit statement of their purpose which was 'the examination of the ever changing doctor/patient relationships, i.e. the study of the pharmacology of the drug 'doctor'.

2.8.2 'The doctor, the patient and his illness'

The Doctor, the Patient and his Illness is the title of Michael Balint's classic book. The work of the Balint groups was controversial and although the groups, in their original form at any rate, are not part of the landscape of medical practice or education today, the impact of this book has been tremendous.

The book, summarising the work of the groups, sets out the simple story that:

- the doctor and the patient developed an emotional relationship during the consultation;
- both doctor and patient had the power to influence the other;
- this power could be used for good or ill;
- collusion can develop between doctor and patient about which problems will be recognised and which will not;
- power flows between doctor and patient.

In this book Balint gives advice on ways in which psychotherapy may be used in either a single consultation or an ongoing series of consultations, but the book is most remarkable for its analysis of the process of diagnosis and the relationship between doctor, patient and illness in the long-term management of chronic health problems.

2.8.3 The apostolic function

Balint's definition of the role of the doctor emphasised the 'apostolic mission or function' which he described by saying that 'it was almost as if every doctor had revealed knowledge of what was right and what was wrong for patients to expect and to endure, and further, as if he had a sacred duty to convert to his faith all the ignorant and unbelieving among his patients.' Patients devised their own techniques for challenging the power of the doctor.

2.8.4 The games patients sometimes have to play

The apostolic function of the doctor is a powerful image but Balint's theories and 'Weltanschauung' were subsequently overtaken, in a move from what was called the psycho-dynamic view of the consultation, to a transactional view of the consultation. Transactional analysis of a social function was developed by <u>Eric Berne</u>, a North American psychiatrist most famous for his books such as <u>*Games People Play*</u> and <u>*What do you say after you say Hello?*</u> and in these books he described social interactions as a game.

The language of game playing is sophisticated and esoteric, for example:

- the initiator starts a game by issuing a 'con', which is an invitation to join in the game;

- the second party joins the game if they have a 'gimmick' i.e. a weakness or a need, and because they have a 'gimmick', they make a response to the 'con.'

The initiator can at any moment shift the whole basis of the game by making what is known as a switch. In the book on <u>Understanding the Consultation</u>, Tim Usherwood gives the following example:

Patient: Do you think I will get better (con)?

Doctor: Of course you will (response).

Patient: That's what you told my neighbour but look how bad she is now (switch).

These games were, however, also described by the British humourist <u>Stephen Potter</u> in his books on one-upmanship and gamesmanship, and parts of those books focus specifically on the doctor/patient relationship, on what he called MD-manship and patientship.

2.8.5 The functions of the consultation

The consultation therefore is a complex negotiation with a number of functions.

- The diagnosis and treatment of disease – the watchmaker function.

- The relief of anxiety – the magical function.

- The validation of illness – the St Peter function.

- Filling out the forms – the bureaucratic function.

As doctors seek to concentrate on the increasingly complex technical task of diagnosis and treatment, other professions are assuming the role of healer.

2.9 The clinician as healer

2.9.1 Curing and healing are not synonyms.

The term 'cure' is relatively specific, as in 'the operation cured the disease'. However the curing of disease is only one part of clinical practice. The process of 'healing' has two broader meanings - intransitive and transitive:

- intransitive healing – a process that the body undergoes, for example 'the wound heals over a two week period';

- transitive healing – an intervention by someone or something which makes the person feel better and may cure the disease.

Healing is particularly relevant to incurable diseases. A disease that is curable by outside intervention is, by definition, finite. However, even where effective treatments are available for chronic diseases and health problems, patients often cannot return to the same level of health they enjoyed before, for example, developing arthritis or multiple sclerosis, or suffering a stroke. The progress of diseases such as these may be halted or slowed, but tissue is irreparably damaged, producing permanent physical effects, sometimes with psychological consequences.

2.9.2 Curing disease and healing suffering

The progress and effects of chronic disease can sometimes be mitigated, but the patient needs help to come to terms not only with persistent symptoms and disability but also with their emotional reaction to these problems.

Many patients feel a sense of injustice, best summarised by the rhetorical question, 'Why me?' This question encapsulates the feelings of anger some individuals may experience when they develop a serious health problem, and it is related to the religious preoccupation with the meaning of suffering, a branch of religious study known as theodicy.

2.9.3 Doctors are more than drugs

In coining the phrase 'the drug (called) doctor', Michael Balint made an important point, but the word 'drug' is so powerfully associated with the concept of cure or symptom control that the phrase 'the drug doctor' does not adequately express the fact that doctors can also be healers by relating properly to patients.

For some clinicians, the emphasis on uncertainty and the promotion of evidence-based medicine pose great challenges in their professional life, as a cry from the heart in *The British Medical Journal* described clearly, because the pre-occupation with the search for evidence may, in the author's view, have reduced the clinician's commitment to the human side of healthcare.

> *Yet, I fear that our search for certain proof has eroded valuable components of care. Taking time with patients, handholding, explaining, comforting, listening, providing hope, and taking interest in our patients' lives are becoming passé in the evidence based revolution of medicine. These lost arts were the mainstay of practice 100 years ago. Our colleagues of past centuries often used foolhardy, unproved, and, occasionally, outright dangerous measures to combat disease before the availability of antibiotics, antidepressants, and antihypertensives.*

> *However, our predecessors often realised the limitations of their medicine and spent time in activities that we no longer esteem because they are not supported by evidence in a peer reviewed publication or the Cochrane Collaboration. We presume that we are better doctors with all of the new tools of science. But I am not so certain. In some aspects we seem to be deficient. With new yardsticks of evidence based medicine we have quickly abandoned vital aspects of medicine that are the most difficult to teach, to measure, and to explain.*[16]

2.9.4 All clinicians can be healers

It is not only doctors who are healers. The nurse is often regarded as a healer within the clinical team, complementing the curative work of the doctor by caring and healing. In adopting this approach, nurses, and members of other professions allied to medicine, sometimes see themselves as offering a holistic approach to the patient's problem. They seek to see the disease in the context of the whole person and to promote healing, whereas doctors, in the opinion of the other clinicians, focus on the disease and not the person. This can cause conflict within the team.

2.9.5 Non-clinicians can be healers

The concept of healing is, of course, long established and in Christian societies Jesus Christ is often portrayed as the first healer. Today many people other than clinicians claim healing powers, from individual 'faith healers' through to members of groups, and practitioners of Christian Science.

2.9.6 Spontaneous healing

The term 'spontaneous healing' is increasingly used to describe the curing of an incurable disease, either without obvious external cause or because of an intervention, for example dietary change. Jerome Groopman describes a case of spontaneous healing in his book *Second Opinions* when a person with incurable and apparently terminal cancer becomes completely free of the disease. Andrew Weil, author and creator of integrative medicine in his book *Spontaneous Healing*, describes a number of cases of people whose incurable diseases vanished.

2.9.7 The elements of healing

Healing may be spontaneous and many people do come to terms well with chronic disease without outside help, but when an outsider, a clinician or non-clinician, tries to promote healing this may be done using one or more of the following methods:

- Talking: encouraging the patient to tell their story in what is now sometimes called 'narrative medicine', based in part on the wonderful work of Arthur Kleinman, Professor of Medical Anthropology at Harvard, whose book *Illness Narratives* describes how a patient's healing can be helped by encouraging him or her to talk.

- Counselling: advising people on techniques they could use to adapt more quickly to their insoluble health problems.

- Touching and holding.

- Praying: for patients with religious beliefs.

- Empathising: the clinician should appear sympathetic and caring and it has been argued that many of the beneficial results of placebos are in fact due to the relationship the patient has with the clinician.

- Listening.

These techniques can be learned, but the skill of the successful healer may be acquired long before he enters professional training because the interventions may be as much a reflection of the healer's personality as the result of training. The healer's influence appears to be mediated by the relationship that develops with the patient, and the need for a new style of practice has been clearly described by one of the people who has studied the work of the physician in most detail, Howard Brady, who wrote

> *In medicine, especially a male-dominated world of medicine, close relationships seem scary and potentially overwhelming, whereas isolation seems safe. Our own sense of safety in emotional distance has probably led us to be overeager to hear the message of detached concern, with the emphasis on the detached rather than the concern. It might be time to explode the myth of getting too close to the patient as a serious danger of attending carefully to the patient's story and affect.* [17]

2.9.8 Narrative medicine

Narrative medicine is a term being used with increasing frequency.

As commonly occurs when a technical term becomes part of everyday language, it is used in different ways by different writers. Writing in the *Annals of Internal Medicine*, one of the world's most important medical journals, Rita Charon defines narrative medicine as medicine 'practiced with the narrative competence to recognize, interpret, and be moved to action by the predicament of others'. She defines five different types of narrative writing in medicine (Table 7). [3]

Table 7: Types of Narrative Writing in Medicine	
Genre	**Example**
Medical Fiction	*How Green is my Valley*, by A.J. Cronin
The Lay Exposition – accounts of decision making written by physicians for the public	*The Blood of Strangers: True stories from the Emergency Room*, by Frank Hyler
Medical Autobiography	*The Story of San Michele,* by Axel Munthe
Stories from Practice – accounts by physicans for other physicians	'The patient who changed my practice' series in the *British Medical Journal*
Writing exercises during medical training	

The term Narrative Medicine is now given to a style of clinical practice which concentrates on taking the patient's experience as an essential foundation for clinical decision-making. Interestingly, one of the best books on the interpretation of the term is the book entitled *Narrative Medicine* by Trish Greenhalgh, one of the leading exponents of Evidence-based Medicine, which is sometimes portrayed as the antithesis to narrative medicine. Both research-based evidence and the patient's narrative are important, but for the healer, the latter may be more important than the former.

2.9.9 The patient as healer

The patient has to be centrally involved in healing and needs to be given the resources to do so.

References

(1)   Kay, H.E.M. (1974) Letter in *The Lancet* ii: 586.

(2)   Foucar, E. (1996) Carcinoma-in-situ of the breast: have pathologists run amok? *The Lancet,* 347: 707-8.

(3)   Sackett D.L., Rosenberg W.M.C., Gray J.A.M., Haynes R.B. and Richardson W.S., (1996). Evidence-based medicine: what it is and what it isn't. *BMJ,* 312: 71-2.

(4)   Sackett, D. L., Straus, S., Richardson, W.S., Rosenberg, W., Haynes, R.B. (1999).Evidence-based Medicine. Harcourt Brace.

(5)   Brett, A.S. (1989) Treating hypercholesterolemia. How should practicing physicians interpret the published data for patients? *New Eng. J. Med.,* 321: 676-9.

(6)   Malenka, D.J., Baron, J.A., Johansen, S., Wahrenberger, J.W. and Ross, J.M. (1993) The framing effect of relative and absolute risk. *J. Gen. Intern. Med.,* 8: 543-48.

(7)   Naylor, C.D., Chen, E. and Strauss B. (1992) Measured enthusiasm: does the method of reporting trial results alter perceptions of therapeutic effectiveness? *Ann. Intern. Med.,* 117: 916-21.

(8)   Hux, J.E. and Naylor, C.D. (1995) Does the format of efficacy data determine patients' acceptance of treatment? *Med. Decis. Making,* 15: 152-7.

(9)   Malenka, D.J., Baron J.A., Johansen, S., Wahrenberger, J.W. and Ross, J.M. (1993).The framing effect of relative and absolute risk. *J. Gen. Intern. Med.,* 8: 543-48.

(10) Forrow, L., Taylor, W.C. and Arnold, R.M. (1992) Absolutely relative: how research results are summarized can affect treatment decisions. *Am. J. Med.,* 92: 121-3.

(11) Bucher, H. and Weinbacher, K.G. (1994) Influence of method of reporting

study results on decision of physicians to prescribe drugs to lower cholesterol concentration. *BMJ*, 309: 761-4.

(12) Fahey, T., Griffiths, S. and Peters, T.J. (1995) Evidence-based purchasing: understanding results of clinical trials and systematic reviews. *BMJ*, 311: 1056-60.

(13) Schwartz, L.M., Woloshin, S., Black, W.C. and Welch, H.G. (1997) The role of numeracy in understanding the benefit of screening mammography. *Ann. Intern. Med.*, 127: 966-72.

(14) Cuddihy, T. (2001) *BMJ*, 323: 460

(15) Kaptchuk, T.J. and Eisenberg, D.M. (2001) A Taxonomy of Unconventional Healing Practices. *Ann. Intern Med.*, 135: 196-204

(16) Rushton, J.L. (2001) The burden of evidence. Personal View. *BMJ*, 323: 349.

(17) Brady, H. (1997) Placebo Response, sustained relationship and emotional resilience in practice. *J. Am. Coll. Family Practice*, 10: 72-74.

(18) Charon, R. (2001) Narrative Medicine: Form, Function and Ethics. *Ann. Intern. Med.*, 134: 83-87.

Section 3

Skills and Resources for Resourceful Patients

In essence, the task of the clinician, as outlined in the previous section, has not changed substantially in the 20th century, and will persist throughout the 21st century. In the former period, however, the clinician had all the resources – the patients simply had to be patient. The 21st century patient needs a number of resources: some are internal – skills and the confidence to use them – others have to be provided for resourceful patients to realise their potential.

3.1 Knowledge
3.2 Skills to appraise knowledge
3.3 Skills for consulting
3.4 Skills for decision-making
3.5 Skills for decision-taking
3.6 Resources – pathways and guidebooks for patient journeys
3.7 Resources for patients – coaching
3.8 Resources for patients – confidence and authority
3.9 Resources – Patient Owned Web Record (POWR)
3.10 Ethical issues in the promotion of the resourceful patient

3.1 Knowledge

It is now recognised that patients need knowledge about their disease and its treatment.

3.1.1 Patient knowledge before the Web

Studies of patients in every culture and country have shown that patients are not ignorant about disease and illness. Patients' knowledge, however, has traditionally been derived from the local community, friends, and family. It is knowledge of a different type to the knowledge that clinicians have.

In the last few decades of the 20th century, the amount of medical knowledge of high quality grew rapidly and became much more relevant to the healthcare problems that patients faced than the beliefs that they had acquired from intermittent contact with the health service and frequent contact with members of their own community. However, when people sought more knowledge, they found they were often excluded from medical libraries. Public libraries, except for the largest, had a slender stock of books on medical subjects, usually consisting only of 'Home Doctor' books, which by and large present a biased, greatly simplified and often out-of-date summary of medical knowledge.

3.1.2 Patient knowledge on the Web

Everything has changed with the World Wide Web and large numbers of Web sites are now available. Famine has turned to surfeit, and although high quality information, such as the abstracts of *Cochrane Reviews*, are available on the World Wide Web, there is also a large amount of junk. Studies of specific topics such as depression or incontinence have revealed that much of the information is misleading, sometimes plain wrong, and occasionally harmful.

Two approaches have been adopted to try to deal with this problem:

- hallmarking the process by which the sites have been developed, for example the <u>BIOME</u> system;

- hallmarking content, as attempted by the <u>Health on the Net Foundation</u>.

These tasks resemble the task faced by Hercules in the Augean stables, and in a *British Medical Journal* editorial provocatively entitled 'Kitemarking the West Wind', [1] <u>Tony Delamothe</u>, who has led the *BMJ*'s excellent Web initiatives, argued that hallmarking was probably an impossible exercise. He cited as evidence the fact that one study conducted in 1998 had shown that there were, even then, 47 different instruments for rating Web sites, none of which had been tested for reliability or validity, with a further 15 instruments appearing between that study in 1998 and the date of the editorial on 7 October 2000. It is certainly important to flag up high-quality sites, but the responsibility can never be taken away from the reader, and for this reason the *Journal of the American Medical Association* came up with the principle of *caveat lector* – let the reader beware.

It is easier if site designers concentrate not only on usability but also on accuracy, using a tool such as <u>DISCERN</u> when creating sites. So far as content is concerned, perhaps the simplest step is to ensure that patients and clinicians have access to the same knowledge.

3.1.3 Clinicians and patients should have a common knowledge resource

Hitherto, sites for the public have been prepared separately from sites for professionals, but this is illogical because:

- 5% of the public are at least as well educated as clinicians;

- most healthcare information is relatively simple, and with a little help, many people can understand quite detailed biological information;

- a patient with one problem can spend a large amount of time reading about that problem, whereas the general practitioner has hundreds of problems to cover;

- patients with a rare disease may come to know more about their, or their child's, disease than their family physician, and rightly so; the family physician may see one case in a career and most of the care may be provided by a highly specialised service.

For all these reasons, it makes no sense to have separate knowledge resources for patients and clinicians. The knowledge resource certainly needs to be made available at a number of different levels, but it could be made available for two different levels of reading, and made available entirely on video for people who cannot read at all.

Similarly, readers could be asked to identify their level of biological knowledge, for example:

- biology up to O level/GCSE, or;

- biology up to A level, or;

- a biology degree.

Every patient and clinician should have access to the same single knowledge resource, and the aim of the <u>National electronic Library for Health</u> (NeLH) is to give clinicians and patients full and equal access to the same resource. It recognises that patients will usually wish to use <u>NHS Direct Online</u> first, but in principle patients and clinicians must have access to the same resource of best current knowledge.

This is necessary but not sufficient for two reasons.

3.1.4 Knowledge about healthcare quality

The decisions patients make about which treatment to choose, based on research evidence, are of great importance. However, for treatments such as surgical operations in which the skill of the clinician, or the quality of the supportive services, determine the outcome, many patients would also like to know how good the clinicians who plan to treat them actually are.

The first step in the provision of information about the quality of clinical practice took place when New York State made the outcomes of cardiac surgery in different hospitals available to the public, albeit only after the *New York Times* had forced them to do so. The result was that those hospitals with the worst results, usually hospitals which were doing the fewest operations, stopped doing cardiac surgery. In the United Kingdom, information about heart surgery mortality was published for the first time in 2001, with promises of similar data for other operations and services, to help patients decide which hospital to choose.

The interpretation of data is not straightforward, however; surgeons with low death rates may be operating on less severely ill patients, for example. Furthermore, the position of a hospital on a league table can change from time to time, particularly where the numbers of treatments are small; unpalatable though it may be, one-half of clinicians will always be below average, not because care is substandard but because of the statistical facts of life which mean that one-half of any group will always be below average.

In November 2001, *The Times* published in five instalment its 'hospital consultants guide…in association with PPP Healthcare,' and compiled by Dr Foster, 'an independent company which provides authoritative information about healthcare providers in the UK'. The guide lists consultants with their qualifications and special interests. Some guides also identify some as 'experts' with 'an exceptional record for publishing research in academic journals about their area of interest', but, as yet, publish no figures about the outcome of their treatments.

3.1.5 Necessary but not sufficient

Some patients do not want access to the type of knowledge that is valued by clinicians: they view clinical epistemology as reductionist and positivist and prefer different ways of looking at health and disease. Patients will therefore always want other sources of knowledge.

Knowledge alone will not create the resourceful patient. Patients also need skills.

3.2 Skills to appraise knowledge

Providing knowledge to patients is necessary but not sufficient on its own.

Not all information is of equal quality, and although many patients are rightly willing to accept the clinician's assurance that his knowledge is good enough for the decision they face, the resourceful patient may wish to make his own assessment of the quality of the knowledge that he has been given.

3.2.1 Is the knowledge fit for the purpose?

The patient and the clinician have to decide if the knowledge is fit for the purpose. The quality of knowledge needed to decide whether or not to rub an aqueous cream or a proprietary, more expensive, skin lotion on a patch of dry skin on the dorsal surface of the left wrist is obviously lower than the quality of knowledge required by the patient facing a serious operation or intensive chemotherapy. Just how far a resourceful patient can go is elegantly described by <u>Stephen Jay Gould</u>, a noted palaeontologist, who gives a dramatic account of his appraisal not only of the knowledge he was given by the clinician but also of the quality of the knowledge he found in the literature.

3.2.2 Everyone is being taught to appraise sources of knowledge

1066, 1815, 664, 1314: the proportion of the population able to say what happened on those dates will diminish as the learning of dates is replaced by the appraisal of sources, even in primary school history. Thus the patient in future will have been taught to distinguish between primary and secondary sources and will also know the need to be suspicious of all sources, including primary sources. The attitude developed in history lessons will be relevant in the clinic.

At present, patients probably know to trust professional journals such as the <u>*British Medical Journal*</u> and <u>*The Lancet*</u> more than they would trust a newspaper. In future, as patients become better educated, they will learn to place more trust in systematic reviews of primary sources rather than the primary sources themselves.

3.2.3 Patients can appraise the knowledge itself

Hitherto patients have appraised the source of the knowledge, decided whether or not to trust the doctor or, if not, found another more trusted source of knowledge such as the _BMJ_ or the _British National Formulary_, if available in the local library. However, patients will increasingly appraise knowledge itself, either choosing to do so, or being asked to do so, by clinicians wishing to share decision-making and responsibility. To do this they will need skills or access to the skills of others, for example by being able to use checklists for appraising knowledge such as those available on the Web from the _Critical Appraisal Skills Programme_ in Oxford.

3.2.4 Training patients and their representatives

Three types of critical appraisal skills training are already emerging.

General training for all patients. This is poorly developed at present but will become part of the school curriculum. If pupils are taught to appraise sources in history, they should surely also be taught to appraise sources of knowledge in health and social education.

Training for representatives of patients and the public. Instead of public representatives on health service organisation boards accepting what the experts say, critical appraisal training is now regarded as necessary for any public or patient representative appointed to a health service board or working in a voluntary organisation.

Focused critical appraisal skills training. General training is useful, but people need it most urgently when they face serious decisions. One method of preparing a patient for serious decision-making is through coaching, to help him reflect on the consultation.

3.3 Skills for consulting

Many good books are now available to teach consultation skills to young clinicians, and every medical curriculum now includes communication and patient consultation skills at its core. However, it is not the clinician who consults, it is the patient, so surely it is also the patient who needs help to develop these skills.

3.3.1 'La maladie du petit papier'

Clinicians in the middle of the 20th century used to dismiss as neurotic those patients who brought with them a little piece of paper with questions written on it. Whether such patients really needed the reminder, or whether this was just a way of dropping their gaze to give them some confidence for taking the initiative against the great man, is uncertain. '*La maladie du petit papier*' viewed formerly as a source of annoyance or amusement, however, can be regarded as a consulting aid and it is now recognised that the best use is made of the clinician's time if the patient prepares before the consultation.

3.3.2 General consulting skills for patients

Some decisions are relatively straightforward and only require the patient to elicit practical information. The decision to have a cataract operation, for example, is usually a clear-cut one, but this type of decision is rare. When patients are being asked to consider a course of action for a more complex condition and perhaps a riskier treatment, they need to ask a set of questions, such as:

- what is the natural course of this disease?

- what would happen if we did nothing?

- what treatment options are there?

For each treatment option the patient could ask:

- what is the probability that I will benefit?

- how great is the benefit that I can expect – complete cure or simply a reduction of symptoms?

- what is the probability that I will he harmed?

- how severe are the harmful side effects? Is there a chance of dying?

For both benefits and harms, the patient could ask how good the evidence was on which the clinician was basing his advice.

After discussing conventional therapy, the patient may want to push the clinician further by asking:

- what about complementary or alternative treatments – do people try other types of treatment for this problem? If so, what are they?

- what research is taking place at present and could I enter it?

There are, in addition, some other questions which require more confidence, for example 'questions a patient contemplating a laparoscopic cholecystecomy should ask about the operator' in Nenner, Imperator and Will's paper in the *Annals of Internal Medicine*:

- *Was the surgeon formally trained in a recognised program in laparoscopic cholecystectomy?*

- *How many laparoscopic cholecystectomies did he or she do and what were the frequencies and types of complications?* [2]

Patients could also be taught to ask about the clinician's experience and competence, or to ask for a second opinion. The need to help patients not only articulate the questions they want to ask, but also to summon up the courage to do so, is now recognised by the Department of Health. Patients are encouraged to take someone along with them to the consultation, and the Department of Health has started to provide patients with frequently asked questions which they can adopt or adapt for their own use. For example, the Department's Commission for Health Improvement developed, with the UK Audit Commission, 'Ten essential questions patients should ask at different stages of their treatment':

- How quickly will I be seen by a consultant?

- What are my tests for and when will I get the results?

- Is the doctor I will be seeing a recognised cancer specialist?

- Can I seek a second opinion?

- Will my GP be notified of my diagnosis?

- How quickly will treatment start, what will it be like, and what are the side-effects?

- Can I have chemotherapy in my local hospital?

- Who should I contact if I am worried about my diagnosis, treatment or prognosis?

- Who can offer me and my family support afterwards?

- If I am to die, will I be able to die where I want?

Furthermore, to develop and deliver these questions, the government worked in partnership with a patient-driven charity, Cancer BACUP, whose mission is to improve information for patients.

3.3.3 Creating confidence

Exhorting people to change their attitude is often ineffective. More effective is to change behaviour and let attitude change follow.

One way to change behaviour would be for the clinician to initiate the change by handing out a list of questions patients commonly ask before the consultation starts or, even better, hand out both questions and answers to as many of the questions as possible.

It is even possible to generate confidence in asking for a second opinion and Jerome Groopman, in *Second Opinions*, makes his beliefs and attitudes clear.

> *Second and third opinions are customary in cases…when the illness is rare and treatment is unclear. Similarly, second opinions are usual for diseases that are not rare but are life-threatening. Here, available treatments usually have a high risk of debility or even death. Experimental therapies are frequently considered for life-threatening disorders, and an assessment of their side effects and rationale is vital before entering the clinical trial. This is best done by conferring with an expert who is not himself invested in the testing of the drug.*

3.3.4 Second opinions online

The World Wide Web, of course, offers an ideal means of getting a second opinion online. Furthermore, to assist their decision-making, there is evidence that patients are already seeking second, third, fourth or nth opinions both before and after the consultation.

3.3.5 Patients need better understanding of clinical practice

Simply teaching a patient what to say in a consultation has merits, but of greater importance is to help patients develop a better understanding of clinical practice and clinical decision-making in all its diversity and uncertainty. A curriculum for what every patient needs to understand has been proposed, but this would take much longer to achieve than the straightforward teaching of consultation skills.

3.4 Skills for decision-making

> '*It is important to distinguish between decision-making and decision-taking.*'
>
> *Henry Kissinger*

Decisions have to be taken on an individual basis because evidence, whether expressed as raw knowledge or in a guideline, has to be related to the condition of the particular patient and their values (Figure 12).

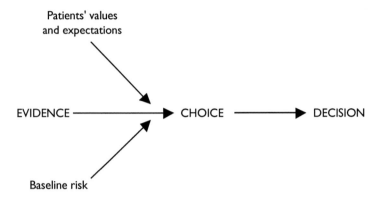

Figure 12

3.4.1 The patient's condition

Research is done on populations, that is, on groups of patients whose members share a single characteristic, for example having a raised level of blood pressure or having breast cancer. However, these patients also vary from one another in many ways, for example by:

- having other risk factors, or

- having other diseases, or

- having a different genetic make-up.

For this reason, information has to be tailored to meet the needs of the individual patient and this is one of the tasks the clinician has to undertake in decision-making. Increasingly, computerised decision support is available to help clinicians and patients relate research findings to individual patients. The <u>National electronic Library for Coronary Heart Disease</u> includes a risk calculator which allows the individual patient's risk factors to be fed into a software system that will produce guidance on their degree of risk.

There has been a surge of interest in computerised decision support systems such as <u>Prodigy</u>, but they have not gained wide acceptance, even when demonstrated as being at least as good as clinicians in making decisions. Part of the reason for this is that they are often less good than clinicians, suitably equipped with best current knowledge at the point of decision-making. For this reason, care has to be taken when appraising new computer decision support systems or when reading articles about them.

3.4.2 Patients' values influence their decisions

The values of the patient have to be taken into account. For example, a patient could be influenced by factors such as the date of birth of their first grandchild, if they are considering intensive chemotherapy with the probability of extending their life expectancy from six months to a year. In such a case, if the chemotherapy appears to give the possibility of surviving to see the grandchild, it might influence them to accept the offer of treatment.

3.4.3 The patient's values and the clinician's values may differ

What is clear is that clinicians and patients have different values, with clinicians giving a higher value to benefit, and patients giving a higher value to the side effects of treatment.

One study showed that clinicians would be willing to offer treatment at a level of blood pressure at which only one person in 100 would benefit, whereas patients would accept treatment at a higher level of blood pressure when one in 33 would benefit. This type of treatment decision is particularly important where there are high stakes to play for, for example at the end of life, and Jerome Groopman's clinical enigma (described on pages 55-6 of *Second Opinions*) illustrates clearly how values can differ between clinician and patient and within one family.

> *'You all understand the events of last night?' I asked. Before sounding out their wishes I needed to be certain everyone was at the same level of knowledge.*
>
> *'I think we do', Jared answered. June and Faith silently nodded. Jared continued: 'and we have real concerns about what is happening.'*
>
> *His face was grim.*
>
> *'What's the point here? Dad has end-stage myelofibrosis. You've got him on a ventilator. He's at a maximum FiO2. His circulation is dependent on a pressor, Levophed. And his creatinine is climbing. Next you'll have to begin dialysis.'*

I glance at June, then at Faith; each wore an uncertain expression. Carolyn looked perplexed.

'Jared was an ICU nurse,' I explained to Carolyn.

3.4.4 C2P decision-making

The main mode of decision-making is clinician to patient – C2P decision-making. This usually takes place within the context of the consultation. Although many clinicians, such as radiologists, make decisions which affect patients without these face to face meetings, the final decision is often taken during or after a consultation. Because consultations are very limited in time and are highly charged emotionally, clinicians are increasingly using decision aids to help patients appraise options and consider the decision. These patient decision aids offer patients information independent of the clinician's message and medium.

3.4.4.1 The clinician's message

When the clinician transmits information there is always a possibility that:

- the information is biased to begin with, or

- the clinician imparts bias to unbiased information.

It is now recognised that the scientific literature on which medicine is based is biased towards a positive and optimistic view of the benefits of medicine for many reasons, such as the desire of journal editors to publish articles with positive findings rather than articles that are inconclusive or negative. Furthermore, it is now known that the way in which many benefits are described in terms of relative risk reduction makes the beneficial effect seem greater than if they were described in terms of the absolute reduction in risk. This phenomenon, which can be observed in clinicians and policy-makers as well as patients, is known as framing.

3.4.4.2 The medium

The medium, the clinician himself, can be as important as the message, and it is known that the following factors influence the consultation, decision-making, and the eventual decision:

- the gender of clinician and patient;

- the race of clinician and patient;

- the age of the patient;

- the class and wealth of the patient.

Even the dress and bearing of the clinician can be important, as Jerome Groopman describes in the story (in <u>Second Opinions</u>) about his first-born son. He was strongly influenced by the appearance of the paediatrician, who

> ... despite the steamy summer heat and the holiday .... wore a starched buttoned-down blue shirt, paisley bowtie and knee-length white coat with his name embroidered in blue script over the left breast pocket. His crisp professional appearance reassured me. In Los Angeles I was disturbed by the indifferent attire of many of the younger doctors: the unkempt hair, running shoes and jeans bordered on sloppiness and did not indicate to the patient the sense of order and attention to detail essential to diagnosis and treatment.

The 'professionally' dressed doctor was unfortunately wrong.

Face to face communication can be complemented by other media, such as a video. For example, in a study of the use of a video before a consultation in which women were being counselled about the risk of breast cancer, the video was acceptable and beneficial. [3]

A systematic review of the research on different methods of giving information to patients with cancer was commissioned by the Department of Health. 120 studies were identified but, using the quality criteria employed in conducting a systematic review, only ten of those studies were considered to provide strong enough evidence to guide policy-makers and clinicians. These high quality studies had examined the effectiveness of:

- audiotapes,

- personalised health record cards,

- booklets,

- videos,

- personalised computer print-outs,

- follow up telephone calls.

The researchers found that the interventions had a positive effect on:

- patient knowledge,

- patients' ability to recall knowledge given previously,

- patient satisfaction with information given.

The authors' conclusion was that these methods of preparing patients for the consultation, and helping them reflect on it, are 'mostly inexpensive and are not time-consuming to introduce into practice'. [4]

Patients can also be given tape recordings of consultations. In a systematic review of eight randomised controlled trials, it was concluded that the provision of written summaries and tape recordings 'helps patients with cancer to remember what was discussed and thus better inform family members'. [5] This practice is now recommended for all consultations about cancer, and for consultations with the parents of seriously ill children.

3.4.5 *Patient to patient consultation*

Patients are also influenced by other patients and this factor is increasingly playing a part in decision-making. Decisions aids now commonly incorporate contributions from patients, and an ambitious project aims to create a database of individual patient experiences (DIPEX) that could be used for education and research and, most important of all, for patients and clinicians to use in decision-making.

In Australia, 'peer leaders' of the same age were used in a programme to educate adolescents with asthma. The effects of this programme were compared with the conventional approach, in which education was provided by clinicians. [6] The effects were significant: compared with the clinician-educated group, the peer-educated group had:

- less time off school;

- fewer asthma attacks;

- better emotional health;

- better physical health;

- better quality of life.

Patient to patient support can be very effective.

3.4.6 Clinician to clinician decision-making

Clinician to clinician decision-making – second opinions – are part of standard medical practice, particularly when the illness is relatively uncommon, and where the clinician's primary responsibility and treatment options are unclear. Patients sometimes find it difficult to ask for a second opinion. However clinicians, in part to share responsibility, will probably increasingly offer to seek a second opinion, and as medicine becomes more complex and specialised, second opinions will also become more prevalent.

3.4.7 Patient to clinician decision-making

What has been described hitherto has been the traditional method of decision-making, with clinicians initiating and directing the debate. Increasingly, however, patients are starting to initiate and direct decision-making and in the remainder of this book we describe how this approach can be promoted and facilitated.

3.5 Skills for decision-taking

As Henry Kissinger emphasised, decision-making lines up the options and sorts out the values, and then comes the crunch – decision-taking.

3.5.1 Each patient has a preferred style

There are different ways of describing the decision-taking style. An American study of women with breast cancer, [7] classified the style into three main types:

- doctor-led,

- patient-shared,

- patient-led.

This study found that:

- 22% wanted to select their own treatment – patient-led;

- 44% wanted a collaborative approach – shared decision-taking

- 34% wanted to delegate responsibility to their clinician – doctor-led.

83

Of particular concern was the finding that there was poor correlation between the preferred style of decision-taking and the way in which the decision was actually taken. Only 42% of women achieved their preferred level of control. Although the patient's preference for style can be matched to that of the doctor, a study in the *British Medical Journal* [8] classified decisions as either 'directed' or 'shared' and with this classification found that 39.8%, or four out of ten patients, wished to have shared decision-making. Importantly, the study concluded that:

> *...although this variation seemed to depend on the presenting problem, age, social class and smoking status, these associations are not absolute, with large minorities in each group. It is therefore not possible to assume what style of decision-making a patient wishes.*

Encouragingly, it was found that:

- the majority of patients who preferred a sharing scenario had a doctor whose style was to share the consultation, and

- the majority of those who preferred a directed scenario had a doctor whose style was directive.

3.5.2 All patients must be given information

Patients who say they do not want an open style of decision-making should nevertheless be offered all the information about treatment options, if for no other reason than that patients sometimes complain or sue when things go wrong, solely on the grounds that they do not recollect being informed about the risks of treatment. In *The Patient* by Michael Palmer, the process of bringing these unpleasant outcomes to the attention of Sara, the patient, before her operation is clearly described:

> *'You may lose the vision in one or both of your eyes.'*

> *'As long as it's only one or both.'*

> *'Okay, then. Initial here... You may lose the use of one or both of your arms.'*

> *'Arms? I mean, really. What do I need arms for, anyhow? Show me one unhappy amoeba. I can scratch my back on a tree like the bears and eat pie like those guys in the county fair.'*

> *'Initial... You may lose the use of one or both of your legs.'*

> *'Jessie, please.'*

'Sara, hospital policy says I have to read this neurosurgery op permit to you out loud, and you know what a policy nerd I am. So stop giving me a hard time and let me finish.'

'Giving you a hard time? It's my damn brain tumour.'

'Touché.'

3.5.3 Reaching agreement on style

When patients become more resourceful, it will become necessary for clinician and patient to agree on how the decision should be taken, because the decision may not even be constant for the one patient, and it is clear that doctors will need both time and skill to determine the style of decision- making preferred by each patient. It is very important to do this because the systematic review of the literature on this subject[9] emphasised that 'some interventions cannot be uniformly introduced into practice without an assessment of informational needs. Evidence indicates that a disparity between information needs and information given can result in patients being more likely to develop affective disorders'.

3.5.4 Resources for action

Once the decision to intervene has been made, the patient needs different types of resources – guidebooks and pathways – to help him find his way to cure and health.

3.6 Resources – pathways and guidebooks for patient journeys

'Have you had your INR, Mr F?'

'What's an INR?'

'It's a blood test for your anticoagulation. We need to know what the state of your blood is before you can have the operation.'

'Well, no-one ever told me I had to have a blood test.'

'Well, Mr F, I'm very sorry but you can't have your operation until you've had the blood test. We'll need to postpone it and rearrange.'

Patients make two types of journey – disease journeys and healthcare journeys. The disease journey progresses through diagnosis to treatment which leads to cure or lifelong co-existence.

The healthcare journey is punctuated by events like consultations, operations and prescriptions, and each journey is unique. The journey may be mundane or fascinating; a new branch of biography – autopathography – was described by Jeff Aronson in the Christmas 2000 edition of the *British Medical Journal* in which he reviewed patients' accounts of their illnesses. However, decisions and events can be identified which are relevant to every patient on a particular journey and to ensure that these are always remembered and that the clinician responds appropriately, guidelines and pathways are developed.

3.6.1 Guidelines and pathways

A guideline presents information to support a decision; a care pathway sets out all the decisions and actions that a clinician and patient should consider, or do, on their journey, or part of their journey.

Care pathways are particularly relevant to discreet parts of the journey, for example:

- going into hospital for hip replacement;
- starting anti-coagulation;
- having a episode of renal dialysis.

Care pathways have been shown to reduce errors and improve the efficiency of care, principally by ensuring that small but significant events are not overlooked by busy professionals carrying out routine tasks and procedures, and who are therefore prone to lapses in concentration.

3.6.2 Guidebooks

Most guidebooks recommend specific tours, city walks spelled out street by street, or rural tours village by village. However, most people use guidebooks in their own way, particularly when there are problems. A study of the management of asthma using the care pathway approach[10] found that many of the patients did not want to feel that they were following a pre-set pathway but did want easy access to help and support when a problem occurred.

3.6.3 Crossroads and signposts on the patient's journey

The group that has done most to develop guidebooks for patient journeys is the Harvard-based group led by Professor Al Mulley and Professor Jack Wennberg.

Mulley and Wennberg have worked for years to develop a style of patient guides involving four main stages in travelling:

- getting ready;

- looking ahead;

- gaining perspective;

- moving forward.

3.6.3.1 Getting ready

The person making a decision has to think about the likely end of the journey, for example the decision to accept an antenatal screening test could finish up with a choice of whether or not to have an abortion. If the woman is implacably opposed to abortion, she should not start on the journey without knowing that abortion is a possible option at the end of it. The health care professionals must make sure they are aware of the end of the journey before the journey begins, but the patient, or, in this case, the pregnant woman, needs to be getting ready for decision-making.

3.6.3.2 Looking ahead

In looking ahead the patient needs to reflect before focusing in on the decision, asking questions such as:

- how healthy am I now?

- what are the options that I face?

- what would happen if I did nothing?

If patients wish to take a decision, they need more detailed focus on options.

3.6.3.3 Gaining perspective

In gaining perspective the patient needs to ask questions such as:

- what are the good outcomes of treatment?
- what is the probability that I will get a good outcome?
- what are the bad outcomes of treatment?
- what is the probability that I will get a bad outcome?
- how do I value both the good and the bad outcomes?

It is then time for the patient to move forward, making the best decision they can in the circumstances, aware of the fact that bad outcomes can follow good decisions.

3.6.3.4 Moving forward

One of the areas where Mulley and Wennberg have developed the journey most clearly is the decision faced by men about whether or not to have a PSA test – a prostate specific antigen test – to detect asymptomatic prostate cancer. They have identified at least fifteen crossroads on the prostate cancer journey, one of which is the decision whether or not to accept the offer of a PSA test. When these men were given adequate information about the options, based on the principles outlines above, a significant proportion declined the offer of a PSA test, emphasising that more information does not always lead to more treatment. [11] In this way, resourceful patients make responsible decisions for themselves and for the health service.

<u>The Foundation for Informed Medical Decision-Making</u> produced two simultaneous interactive decision aids to help patients considering hormone replacement therapy and patients considering prostatectomy with their decisions. The evaluation of these aids were very encouraging, [12] with the authors concluding that 'an interactive multimedia decision aid in the NHS would be popular with patients, reduce decisional conflict, and enable patients to play a more active part in decision-making without increasing anxiety.'

3.6.4 The resourceful patient and the pathway

Patients should be given the same pathway as clinicians, because pathways have been shown to be effective and acceptable. The patient could be given responsibility for parts of the pathway and had Mr F in the vignette at the beginning of this chapter been given responsibility for, and authority to carry out, the INR blood test, he would have had his operation on the day planned. The clinician is meant to be the guardian of the patient, but some patients need coaching to help them cope with their journey.

3.6.5 The expert patient

People who have life-long diseases such as diabetes, for which they claim none of the rights of illness, sometimes refer to their problem not as a disease or an illness but as a condition, something they have to live with and manage with occasional help from a professional. In the United States, where patients have traditionally had to manage more of their care including its payment, self-management programmes have been studied and promoted for many years – for example, in the famous Chronic Disease Self-Management Programme at Stanford. In the United Kingdom a number of initiatives focusing on specific diseases have been developed with the lead being taken by mutual aid societies or patient organisations, as they are sometimes called – for example:

- 'Challenging Arthritis' is the name given to the arthritis self-management course developed by the charity Arthritis Care.

- The Self-Management Training Programme for people with depression was developed by people with manic depression, co-ordinated by the Manic Depression Fellowship.

- A structured self-management programme for people with multiple sclerosis has been developed by the Multiple Sclerosis Society.

The Department of Health produced a report on these approaches to chronic disease management called 'The Expert Patient' and a review of the evidence about the benefit of self-management programmes commissioned for the task force which produced the report concluded that among the obvious benefits were:

- reduced severity of symptoms,

- significantly decreased pain,

- improved life control activity,

- improved resourcefulness and life satisfaction.

Table 8: Evidence for impact of self-management programmes on service use	
Chronic pain Arthritis	Reduction in number of visits to health professionals up to 80% [13, 14]
Arthritis Insomnia Asthma	Reduction in number of general practitioner visits up to 44% [15, 16, 17, 18, 19]
Sickle cell disease Asthma	Reduction in number of hospitalisations (up to 31%) and length of stay (up to 50%) [20, 21]
Insomnia	Reduction in number of visits to specialists by 15% [19]
Sickle cell disease Asthma	Reduction in number of accident and emergency department visits up to 39% [20, 21]

The report made eight specific recommendations, namely:

- to promote awareness and create expectations that patient expertise is central in the delivery of care to people with chronic disease;

- to set up a programme to develop more self-management courses and programmes;

- to identify the barriers to the uptake of self-management in the NHS;

- to integrate user-led self-management into the NHS provision of care;

- to ensure that each primary care trust has arrangements for user-led self-management programmes;

- to expand the practical support for user-led programmes;

- to change professional training so that they understand how they can support self-management;

- to establish a national co-ordinating and training resource to promote and realise the concept.

The expert patient with the chronic disease will not need a guide in future. Patients will find their own way to better health.

3.6.6 The need for interpreters

The sight of two world leaders facing each other across a table, each with an interpreter at their elbow, emphasises that without interpretation, dialogue is sometimes impossible when two people meet. The need for interpretation is also common when the patient and clinician are in a consultation.

Sometimes the patient can take an interpreter to the consultation, particularly when the first language of clinician and patient are not the same. An interpreter is, however, also necessary for many consultations when both clinician and patient share the same first language. The interpreter may have to:

- explain the meaning of anatomical terms such as gall bladder or carcinoma *in situ*;
- clarify the options that are on offer to the patient and the consequences, both good and bad, of the options;
- support the patient who feels too timid to ask questions or challenge the clinician, namely act as the patient's advocate as well as interpreter.

Many more patients would like an interpreter present in the consultation than there are interpreters available. To fill the gap, the Department of Health set up <u>NHS Direct</u>, but there are many other services of interpretation provided by voluntary organisations. There are now hundreds of help lines covering both <u>common long-term medical conditions</u> such as rheumatoid arthritis, and rare conditions, such as the service provided by <u>Contact a Family</u>, a charity which provides support and advice for parents who have children with disabling diseases, some of which are so rare that even the paediatrician they are seeing may see a case no more than once a decade.

Even if the first language of the patient and the clinician is the same, interpretation may be necessary. A study of the language used in consultations showed that, to paraphrase Winston Churchill's famous dictum, the Britons and Americans were two nations divided by a common language. The fact that clinician and patient both use English does not mean that each understands the other.[22] Furthermore, the words used act not only as tools to aid diagnosis or clarify options but also as tools of social control, maintaining the power of the doctor over the patient. Often the clinicians used words with the intention of reassuring the patient and reducing their anxiety, but the use of comforting words such as 'it's just a little lesion' not only fail to comfort every patient but also maintain the paternalistic relationship with the clinician as parent and the patient as child. In the 21st century, both clinicians and patients have to view each other as adults.

3.7 Resources for patients – coaching

Boris Becker changes coaches in search of success.

Newspaper headline

Coach:
Convey in or provide with a coach. (1612)
Prepare for an examination; to prime with information. (1849)

Shorter Oxford English Dictionary

Knowledge and skills are sufficient for some people to cope with a consultation; others need coaching to make the best use of their resources in the consultation and in clinical decision-making.

3.7.1 Training and coaching

The job of the *trainer* is to improve the fitness of the individual to ensure that an individual performs as well as possible when under pressure. A high level of fitness is a necessary prerequisite to success, and the provision of coaching does not reduce the need for the individual to acquire knowledge and skills. However, the *coach* focuses much more on the psychological preparation of an individual for a specific event. Many people can be trained how to find knowledge and given the skills to ask questions of clinicians, but coaching increases the probability that the individual will use the knowledge and skills in the crucial consultation.

3.7.2 The crucial consultation

Every consultation is crucial but the experienced clinician becomes accustomed to crucial decisions, for example about which treatment to choose for colorectal cancer, in which he may participate hundreds of times in his career. For the patient, however, familiarity with the crucial consultation is important for they may only have one consultation in which to make a crucial decision and, for many medical problems, that crucial consultation will occur only once in a lifetime. There is increasing interest in coaching patients to prepare them for the consultation.

3.7.3 The benefits of coaching

Coaching primes and prepares the patient. Sportsmen and women choose a coach to help them realise their potential, and coaches do this by:

- rehearsal with feedback – the individual can practise a particular move or sequence of moves time after time to become familiar with the moves, with errors being corrected through feedback;

- preparing for the unfamiliar – the coach helps the person imagine what is going to happen;

- building an inner picture – the coach helps the person he is coaching to develop a clear picture of how they are appearing and behaving. The coach can help individuals get a clear picture of how they should behave in any situation they have never previously encountered;

- psyching up or calming down – some people need to have their confidence built up before a sporting event or consultation to help them believe that they are resourceful, competent and able to ask the questions that they want to ask. Other people need to be calmed down, or they may become too tense, and freeze.

3.7.4 Coaching provides focused preparation

There are different ways in which groups like <u>Health Dialog</u> provide coaching.

- On paper: the simplest form of coaching to help the individual ask the right questions is a leaflet written specifically for the patient to read and practise from before the consultation.

- Web-based resource: interactive Web pages can provide an experience almost like a personal coach, helping the individual prepare for the consultation and formulate the right questions.

- Telephone coaching: new services are developing to allow individuals to prepare for a consultation by discussing options with a coach who not only gives information about different options, to allow them to make an informed choice, but who also helps them prepare intellectually and psychologically for the consultation.

- Face-to-face coaching: general practitioners often perform the function of a coach, helping the individual prepare for their visit to the clinic.

Coaches also help people by reflecting on their performance, both to assist them to come to terms with disappointment and to help them prepare for the next time they may face the same challenge.

3.7.5 Healthcare organisations can encourage coaching

Healthcare organisations of the 21st century should encourage coaching so that patients can make the best use of their limited contact with the service. They can do this by:

- providing learning resources that individuals can use before they come to the clinic, and

- developing their own Web site so that the patient can obtain specific information about the service they are going to encounter.

3.8 Resources for patients – confidence and authority

'I can't understand it, Mr S. You should have had a colonoscopy before coming in for the operation.'

'Well, here I am. This is the day for my operation, and no-one told me I needed a colonoscopy.'

'Well, I'm very sorry but we'll have to put the operation off. The doctor won't want to go ahead without a colonoscopy.'

Many patients are accustomed to managing much more complicated processes than ensuring that they have a colonoscopy before coming to hospital for an operation, so why not give them the authority to do so?

3.8.1 Lean systems

One of the revolutions introduced by <u>lean thinking</u>, usually called 're-engineering' in healthcare, is the need to reduce the number of steps in any process. The more steps there are, for example, in arranging an x-ray, the greater the cost, the more the delay and the higher the probability of error. Patients should therefore be given the authority and ability to organise more of their care. If thousands of people can arrange complicated holidays in lands where they do not speak the language, surely it is possible for a patient to arrange a chest x-ray, a blood test, or a sequence of visits preparatory to an operation.

Mr S is told that he needs a bowel operation. He is asked if he wants to arrange the work-up himself. He says he does because he has a complicated work diary and is travelling in the next few weeks. He is e-mailed the digital care pathway which sets out all the tasks he is required to undertake, and all the contact telephone numbers he needs. He is also given the authority to take whatever action is necessary.

2005 Vignette

3.8.2 Authority

Being given authority is one thing: having the confidence to exercise it is another. If, however, the patient wishes to accept the authority not only for decision-making but also for arranging those parts of his care that are more efficiently arranged by the individual, the health service, and to be specific, the clinicians the patient encounters, have to treat him with respect. The experience of achievement in a friendly environment will build confidence in a way that exhortation will not.

3.8.3 The symbol of authority

The symbol of a patient's authority should be the ownership of his health records.

3.9 Resources – Patient Owned Web Record (POWR)

'I've got breast cancer and ovarian cancer. I've got records in Morecambe Royal Infirmary, the Christie Hospital, the Whittington Hospital and in my general practitioner's surgery. My GP's very good but my records have been mislaid for the last three and a half months. I don't see how it's possible for me to have good care.'

A 72-year-old patient

Healthcare is becoming more:

- complex;
- specialised;
- bureaucratic.

As a consequence, the size of the patient record increases inexorably. Paper records are only effective if the patient is getting all his care in one setting. The simplest solution to this problem is to make the patient the record holder.

3.9.1 Patient-held records

Patient-held records have been shown to be effective in certain relatively simple situations, for example maternity records or child health records. However, the time has now come to create a ubiquitous single record by putting the record of an individual patient on the World Wide Web. Health Level 7 (HL7) standards, an internationally agreed protocol, allow every healthcare organisation to communicate with the Patient Owned Web Record – all that is needed is a commitment to co-operate.

3.9.2 Web-held records

Many companies now offer templates for Web-held records. The technology is simple, but the main concern is security. Encryption allows high levels of security, but any level of security can be cracked by the skilled and determined hacker. However, routinely hacking into people's medical files would not be particularly attractive for the skilled hacker because most medical records are dull. Hackers might be interested in certain types of medical records, for example an access to the medical record of the Prime Minister or in finding out who was infected with HIV, but in estimating the risk of these events it is essential to bear in mind that our current record systems cannot be assumed to be particularly safe. In many hospitals, it is still possible simply to phone a ward and be given information about a person's state of health without a security check.

3.9.3 Ownership

Nobody owns the World Wide Web, but who would own a patient's record on the Web? At present the principle is that the provider of care owns the paper record, but the most effective way of managing a Web record is for the patient to own it. Again fears have been raised about this principle. One of the fears that has been expressed about the Web record is that the patient might tamper with the record to create a case for litigation.

3.9.4 Web records are inevitable

In the UK, the government's *Information for Health* strategy gave a commitment to provide electronic patient records for people receiving care and an electronic health record that would be linked to an individual for life. Change has started, and by 2010 Web records will be ubiquitous. The patient who wants good care should campaign for a Web record as soon as possible.

3.9.5 PING (Personal Internetworked Notary and Guardian Project)

The PING (Personal Internetworked Notary and Guardian Project) at the Boston Children's Hospital has come closest to realising this vision and the aim is to create a patient-owned record with six characteristics:

- comprehensiveness;

- accessibility from work, home and on holiday, as well as the clinic;

- inter-operability with every healthcare organisation;

- confidentiality;

- accountability – changes to the record should be recorded and visible to the patient;

- flexibility, to allow the patient to contribute to research or education.

The PING research team identified two problems and offered them solutions to them (Table 9).

Table 9: Problems and Solutions	
Problem	**Solution**
Health care organisations work in isolation	Record systems should be designed so that they can show all the data using public standards
Patients are increasingly anxious about privacy	Patients should have the control over access to their records

Mandl, Szolovits et al, BMJ [23]

The electronic medical record should be:

- comprehensive and cover all aspects of health;
- accessible everywhere;
- interoperable with all healthcare systems;
- confidential and private;
- open to the patient's scrutiny.

The key issue is confidentiality, but the present system of patient records is by no means secure, and even though many people will move money on the Internet, fears of the misuse of medical information are more deeply-rooted. Perhaps the best approach would be to make the electronic record a right in the first instance so that those patients who believed their care could be safer and better by the use of electronic medical records need not have their rights impaired by those patients who understandably fear the Internet.

3.10 Ethical issues in the promotion of the resourceful patient

In many countries the improvement in health of the whole population has been accompanied by a widening health gap between the social classes with most wealth and those with least wealth. This widening gap reflects broad social trends, with the new style economy polarising those at the very bottom of the pecking order, having not only the lowest wages but also the greatest insecurity. Furthermore, in a knowledge society, decisions which are knowledge-based will be better made by those who are better educated, and they are usually those who are better paid. Similarly, knowledge resources made available to all patients would probably be adopted more frequently by better educated and wealthier people who already have access to more material resources. It is important, therefore, in promoting a range of measures to give patients more power, that these measures do not further widen the health gap.

3.10.1 Not providing resources is no option

One approach would be to continue as before, with all patients equally dependent and powerless, but this option is unacceptable. Even if only 5% of the population wish to hold their own records and manage much of their care, there is sufficient justification for them to be allowed to do so. At present change takes place at the rate of the slowest mover, and if some people are so anxious that they do not wish their health record to be on the Web, that should not prevent those who want to do so from achieving their objective.

What we are arguing, however, is not simply that 5% be allowed to have the necessary resources, but that the basic premise should be that individual patients hold their own records, organise their care and take responsibility, provided, of course, they are given the skills and resources to do so. This premise, if it were adopted, would be a change in the clinical paradigm and the result would be that those who did not choose to acquire the skills and use the resources would be regarded as deviant, even if they were in the majority. This could widen the health gap. However, there is no option but to offer skills and resources, and we must therefore compensate for individuals or sub-groups within the population who might have particular difficulty in coping with the new system. Groups worthy of particular consideration are:

- people with a learning disability;

- people who become incompetent because of brain disease;

- young people who become incompetent because of brain injury or assault;

- children and adolescents.

This is, of course, already an issue[24] and those who have problems with reading are at a disadvantage. One study found that 'people with limited reading ability have poorer health outcomes'[25]. The World Wide Web, however, does offer opportunities for solving, or at least mitigating the problem because it is much easier, and cheaper, to make and present multi-media versions of printed patient education material, such as incorporating sound and video clips in different languages. The technology that could in one sense widen the health gap, could also help to narrow it.

3.10.2 People with a learning disability

In a world in which shared decision-making and evidence-based patient choice are promoted, people with a learning disability could be at a disadvantage, because they have been regarded as not needing to be provided with the opportunity to make decisions.

Although it is sometimes necessary for action to be taken that is against the express wish of the person with a learning disability, the basic premise must be that the person with a learning disability should have the same rights as other patients and, in consequence, to adapt decision-making in such a way that people with a learning disability are empowered. This issue was addressed by the <u>NHS Breast and Cervical Screening</u> Programmes, when women with learning disabilities and staff working with them were concerned that the information issued by the screening programmes did not take into account the fact that people with a profound learning disability might be unable to understand the language in which the choices were being offered to them.

Based on this experience, the National Screening Committee agreed the following measures:

- each national screening programme should develop good practice frameworks in order to achieve equity of access for people with learning disabilities.

- performance management mechanisms should be used to ensure that such frameworks are in place and are adhered to;

- health professionals who work with people with learning disabilities should ensure that understanding of screening programmes is included in general education about healthcare for this population.

The Cancer Screening Programmes set up a special project, involving women with learning disabilities, to discuss the issues and develop educational material that would allow people to make informed choices, and the general principles that emerged from this project were that wherever possible, women with a learning disability should:

- *have access to information to enable them to make their own decisions about whether or not to accept the invitation to attend for breast screening or cervical screening;*

- *know what to expect when they attend for screening so that it is a positive experience;*

- *understand the possible consequences of screening and the need to be aware of changes in their own bodies.*

3.10.2.1 Preparing good quality information

The women with learning disabilities developed materials, both in simple language and in pictures, to allow people with limited reading ability to comprehend the options that were being presented to them. When this material was examined by the National Screening Committee it became obvious that it was very good, not only for people with a profound learning disability, but also for people who had difficulty with reading, a significant proportion of the population. One outcome of the project was the decision that the picture leaflet and the simple invitation letter should be sent to all women who had not previously responded to an invitation to come for screening (sometimes classified as 'refusers'), acknowledging the fact that a proportion of those women had not responded simply because they did not understand the letter of invitation.

3.10.2.2 Changing the system

People are not only empowered by clearer words and better understanding. Healthcare systems have to change to facilitate and support empowerment, both at the point of decision about whether or not to have a mammogram or cervical smear and when actually attending for mammography or the smear test. Shown in the table below is an example of the good practice advice given to ensure that once a decision had been made, further issues could be adequately discussed so that women with learning disability would feel that they were being empowered during the process as well as during the invitation (Table 10).

Table 10: Good practice in screening
Book a longer appointment (at the static unit).
If a supporter, friend or relative is due for breast screening at about the same time, it may be helpful to book the screening appointment at the same session.
If possible, provide dedicated time and space for those women who find it difficlut to comply with the social expectations of a waiting room.
Check that the supporter who will accompany the woman understands the screening process and if necessary arrange for a preliminary visit.
Discuss issues of consent with the supporter.
Consider suitability for mammography and seek advice from the radiographer on what is technically possible for women with a physical disability.
Ask the GP or care home to arrange suitable transport for the woman if required.

All these measures increase the probability that the person with the learning disability will be able to use the resources developed for them.

3.10.3 People who become incompetent because of brain disease

People with learning disability have impaired power of communication, and sometimes reasoning, but at least they are stable. More common and more complicated are the problems posed by people who lose the power of communication and who may or may not have advocates who can speak on their behalf.

3.10.3.1 Terminal incapacity

The patient is wheeled into the emergency room; blood pressure has collapsed and the patient is unconscious, barely alive. The team, usually consisting of young doctors and nurses, swings into action, a central venous line is put in, fluids are given, the position is stabilised and the diagnosis made. During the course of the assessment, the presence of a long-standing stroke with severe disability is detected. Then some more details arrive and it turns out that the patient also has Alzheimer's Disease, lives alone, and has no relatives. Four days later, there is no sign of improvement and more intensive measures are necessary; infection sets in and intravenous antibiotics are required.

This scenario is common and young doctors and nurses have little option but to intervene when an old person is brought in; if they do not, they could be accused of ageism or even manslaughter. Furthermore, decisions about stopping or withholding treatment, even after the initial breathless emergency is over, can also lead to problems for the medical staff, and the letters NFR or DNR, 'not for resuscitation' or 'do not resuscitate', are now unacceptable.

In these circumstances there is increasing interest, particularly in the United States, in the Living Will or 'instructive Advance Directive'.

3.10.3.2 An instructive Advance Directive – You Decide

You Decide is the name of a book by Evelyn J. Van Allen on 'easing Living Wills and other Advance Directives to guide your treatment choices'. The book gives clear and explicit advice on the preparation of an Advance Directive and covers the various changes that are required, depending upon the particular state in which the person is living. The guidance is explicit and an example of the type of options that are provided in the book is provided. A Directive is written and signed and can even be videotaped, but of course merely preparing an Advance Directive does not guarantee that it will be used, and one study showed that only 26% of patients who previously made an Advance Directive had that Living Will recognised during their hospital stay. The importance of the Advance Directive was also revealed by this study because when it was found and identified, it appeared to influence treatment decisions in 12 out of 14 cases[26].

3.10.3.3 *Public attitudes to Advance Directives*

702 people from Boston, Massachusetts, were included in a survey of attitudes towards life-sustaining treatment and Advance Directives. 297 either refused or were ineligible for one reason or another, leaving 405 patients in the survey, to which were added 102 members of the general public. 93% of those patients interviewed, and 89% of members of the general public said that they wished to have an Advance Directive. The authors concluded that 'Advance Directives, as part of a comprehensive approach such as that provided by a Medical Directive, are desired by most people, require physician initiative, and can be achieved during a regular office visit'.[27]

3.10.3.4 *Evidence-based Advance Directives*

The Advance Directive sounds like a good resource, but of course at the end of life, circumstances are not generalisable and each case has its own individual particularities. Furthermore, it may be many years since the patient wrote the Advance Directive and his views may have changed in the interim.

For example, in an Advance Directive patients, or potential patients, are asked to indicate whether or not they want 'mechanical breathing (respiration by machine through a tube in the throat) or dialysis (cleaning the blood by machine or by fluid passing through the belly)'. In a study of the wishes of 186 patients in the United States, the possible future need for mechanical breathing or, to be more precise, 'intubation and ventilatory support', was assessed by explaining what would happen during a severe pneumonia and what would be involved in intubation and ventilatory support. Nearly all the patients given this information said that would want intubation and ventilatory support and the more information they received, the more likely were they to accept the offer or be prepared to tolerate it for longer periods of time. These authors concluded that their study suggested that giving more detailed information about a particular medical problem or intervention 'may have strong effects on the preference of patients and their willingness to accept or refuse invasive medical interventions'.[28]

Unfortunately this type of decision often has to be made for patients who would never think of making an advance directive – people severely injured by accident or assault.

3.10.4 People who become incompetent because of brain injury or assault

Decisions to continue or withdraw treatment from someone who is going to die in the near future, often at the end of a long life, are harrowing. Even more difficult are decisions about intensive intervention, which carry a significant risk of aggravating the injury to the brain, for severely ill younger patients. This problem occurs frequently in places where young men are admitted with gunshot injuries to the head and

- where the outcome of surgical intervention could be:

- recovery, either complete or with some residual disability,

- death;

- survival in a vegetative state.

Furthermore, the two adverse outcomes, death and survival in a vegetative state, may be sub-divided into outcomes as listed below:

- death, when the patient would have survived but in a vegetative state if he had not had surgery;

- survival after surgery in a vegetative state when the patient would have died if he had not had surgery;

- survival in a vegetative state when the patient would have had a better outcome, e.g. survival with minor disability, if he had not had surgery.

In one study of this group of patients, the authors found that the Glasgow coma scale, which is a method of determining the depth of brain damage, allowed relatives and clinicians to 'limit the number of pointless neurosurgical procedures' but they emphasised that any guidelines developed should favour those who had even a small chance of living independently[29]. The authors of this study recognised that it was carried out at a time when 'public health care dollars are increasingly scarce' and emphasised the need to be aware of this so that any decision should not be taken on the basis of cost or prognosis alone, but that ethical issues should always be involved, with the physician's role being as 'a provider of information and core decision-maker'.

3.10.4.1 Are Advance Directives much use in empowering patients who are temporarily disempowered?

Advance Directives are receiving increased publicity. Their impact has hitherto been limited, particularly because even when they have been written, they may not be found when required. Furthermore, for young people with severe illness or injury, Advance Directives are irrelevant because they have rarely been made.

One approach is to train physicians to be sensitive to the options that exist and to develop services so that patients' relatives are empowered to make the decisions that match the patient's values at the end of life, or when difficult decisions are being faced. This approach has largely been used in the hospice movement which itself developed to empower patients at the end of their lives so that they could choose an active approach towards symptom control as opposed to the active approach towards cancer control. The latter was often the only option considered by staff or put to patients in the era before palliative medicine became a recognised and valued branch of medicine.

The growth of the hospice movement world-wide demonstrates how a new environment could create a new culture, and the relevance of the work of the hospice movement to the culture of general hospital care is now recognised[30]. Furthermore, a review of trials of interventions designed to change clinical care at the end of life, which found 16 studies that met explicit criteria for study quality, concluded that it was possible to increase the incorporation of patient preferences in decision-making and that 'intensive educational interventions for physicians and broad educational programmes seem more promising than Advance Directives' in improving the quality of care and the empowerment of patients at the end of life[31].

3.10.4.2 Resourceful patients in intensive care

At the moment of entry to intensive care, the patient is usually unable to play much of a part in decision making, or in their own care. The patient may be unconscious or paralysed and have no relatives or friends to act as advocate. The patient who leaves intensive care alive usually has better physical and psychological function, but is rarely able to use the resources described in this book. Evidence has emerged in 2001 that patients would, on average, benefit from a longer stay in intensive care. A proportion of the patients who die after discharge would not do so if the stay in intensive care were prolonged, but discharge is usually precipitated by the pressure to admit someone else who is in more urgent need of a bed. The staff do not know that the patient they are transferring to a non-intensive care ward will die, but they are often concerned that the patient is discharged too early.

If the patients being discharged could manage all the resources available, they could argue that they should stay longer in intensive care, but there is a limit to what can be expected of even the most resourceful of patients when they are severely ill.

3.10.5 Children

Parents and guardians have the right to make informed choices for children. At Bristol Royal Infirmary, an enquiry following a series of deaths among children with congenital heart disease, focused on informed consent as an issue as important as the competence of the clinicians. This enquiry, whose recommendations on respect, openness and honesty are of great importance, also raised the issue of parents' rights after the death of a child. Parents making decisions on behalf of children, like patients making decisions for themselves, need to know not only about the effectiveness of the intervention but also about the experience of the operator in carrying out that particular intervention.

The American Patients' Association lists five questions that patients or parents could ask of clinicians – provided, of course, that they had the confidence to do so – and although these questions do not relate to children, the principle, and the style of questions, could be used by parents.

- Is the surgeon Board certified?

- Does the surgeon have hospital privileges to do open cholecystectomy?

- Was the surgeon formally trained in a recognised programme in laparoscopic cholecystectomy?

- How many laparoscopic cholecystectomies did s/he do and what were the frequency and types of complication?

The Department of Health's response to Professor Kennedy's inquiry into children's heart surgery at the Bristol Royal Infirmary, emphasised that parents should be 'fully engaged' in decisions about their child. All the points made in the Kennedy Report about the need to communicate openly and honestly with parents and the need to respond truthfully to patients' questions 'be they adult or child' is recognised, reinforcing the point made in the Reference Guide to Consent for Examination and Treatment about the child's right to ask questions.

3.10.5.1 *Going against the wishes of parents*

Occasionally it is necessary for a health service to take the place of parents and make decisions for a child. Among the most dramatic cases are those in which a child, whose parents are Jehovah's Witnesses, requires a blood transfusion. In these cases, the rights of decision-making have to be removed from the parents and transferred to the state, so that an appropriate decision can be made.

3.10.5.2 *Adolescence – a time of transition*

> *Mary X moved from the paediatric diabetic clinic to the adult clinic at the age of sixteen; she was happy for her parents to continue to come to consultations with her.*

> *Mary Y moved from the paediatric diabetic clinic to the adult clinic at the age of sixteen; from that time on she did not want her parents to come to the clinic.*

In healthcare, as in family life, adolescence is a time of negotiation, and resourceful adolescents may wish to assume full responsibility for their care even though, or perhaps because, their parents feel they are not mature enough to do so.

The Department of Health guidelines on seeking consent specifically identify 'young people aged 16-17' as an age group entitled to consent to their own medical treatment. Children under sixteen can also give consent if they have the capacity to 'understand fully what is involved in a proposed intervention', and the level of understanding will obviously vary from one child to another, and be influenced by the complexity of the procedure or options.

3.10.6 Informed consent

Even touching a patient can be regarded as assault if the patient has not given valid consent. Clinicians have to seek consent in a wide variety of different circumstances, for example:

- I am going to touch you in the course of examining you to find out what is wrong with you.

- I am going to take a blood sample from you.

- I am going to insert some stitches in this open wound and wish to explain to you what is going to happen.

- There are two options for treatment: either an operation or drug treatment, and I am going to describe the risks and benefits of each option to you.

In 2001, the Department of Health published a 'Reference Guide to Consent for Examination or Treatment', recognising that the wide range of guidance that had been issued to clinicians was in need of clarification and simplification. Furthermore, the European Human Rights Acts required the United Kingdom to re-visit its legal principles relating to informed consent. The guidance covers a wide range of different situations including seeking consent from adults without capacity, either permanent or 'fluctuating', and children and young people. Specific guidance is given on withdrawing and withholding life-prolonging treatment for both adults and children, again with separate advice given for those without capacity.

The issue of capacity is of central importance, and the Department of Health defines capacity by saying that 'for a person to have capacity he or she must be able to comprehend and retain information material to the decision, especially as to the consequences of having or not having the intervention in question, and must be able to use and weigh this information in the decision making process.' The guidance tries to define 'sufficient information' but the definition provided has a degree of circular logic because it says 'in considering what information to provide, the health professional will try to ensure the patient is able to make a balanced judgement on whether to give or withhold consent.' It specifically advises clinicians to inform the patient of any 'material' or 'significant' risks in the proposed treatment, any alternatives to it, and the risks associated with doing nothing. The General Medical Council states that the doctor should not only do his best in summarising the evidence about treatment options. It requires him also to seek to find out the patient's individual needs and priorities when providing treatment options, because even advice which seems relatively simple has to take into account the condition and values of the individual.

A professor of medical law, commenting on these guidelines, emphasises that 'disclosure of risk is one of the few remaining areas of uncertainty' but concludes that 'patient autonomy has triumphed and people may now decline medical treatment for whatever reason they choose'[32].

References

(1) Delamothe, A., (2000) 'Kitemarking the West Wind'. *BMJ*, 321: 843-844

(2) Nenner, R.P., Imperato, P.J., and Will, T.O. (1994) Questions patients should ask about laparoscopic cholecystectomy. *Ann. Intern. Med.*, 120: 443.

(3) Cull, A., Miller, H., Porterfield, T., Mackay, J., Anderson, E.D.C., Steel, C.M. and Elton, R.A. (1998) The use of videotaped information in cancer genetic counselling: a randomized evaluation study. *Brit J. Cancer*, 77: 830-7.

(4) McPherson, C.J., Higginson, I.J. and Hearn, J. (2001) Effective methods of giving information in cancer: a systematic literature review of randomised controlled trials. *J. Pub. Health Med.*, 23: 227-34.

(5) Scott, J. T., Entwistle, V. A., Sowden, A. J., and Watt, I. (1999) Recordings of summaries of consultations may help patients with cancer. In *The Cochrane Library*, Oxford, Update Software.

(6) Shah, S., Peat, J.K., Mazurski, E.J., Bruce, C., Henry, R.C., Gibson, P.G. (2001) Effect of peer led programme for asthma education in adolescents. *BMJ*, 322: 585-7.

(7) Degner, L.F., Kristjonson, L.J., Bowen, D., Soan, J.A., Camore, K.C., O'Neil, J., Bilodeau, B., Watson, P. and Mueller, B. (1997) Information needs and decisional preference in women with breast cancer. *JAMA*, 277: 1485-92.

(8) McKinstry, B. (2000) Do patients wish to be involved in decision making in the consultation? A cross sectional survey with video vignettes. *BMJ*, 321: 867-71.

(9) McPherson, C.J., Higginson, I.J. and Hearn, J. (2001) Effective methods of giving information in cancer: a systematic literature review of randomised controlled trials. *J. Pub. Health Med.*, 23: 227-34.

(10) Jones, A., Dill, R., and Adams, S. (2000) Qualitative study of views of health professionals and patients on guided self-management plans for asthma. *BMJ*, 321: 1507-10.

(11) Flood, A.B., Wennberg, J.E., Nease, R.F., Fowler, J.F., Ding J. et. al. (1996) The importance of patient preference in the decision to screen for prostate cancer. *J Gen Intern Med.*, 11: 342-349.

(12) Murray, E., Davis, H., Tai, S.S., Coulter, A., Gray, A. and Haines A. (2001) Randomised controlled trial of an interactive multimedia decision aid on hormone replacement therapy in primary care. *BMJ*, 323: 490-3

(13) Davis, R.M., Wagner, E.G. and Groves, T. Editorial in Special Edition of *BMJ* on managing chronic diseases, 7234: 26 February 2000.

(14) National Survey of NHS Patients: General Practice in 1998. NHS Executive, 1999.

(15) Erens, B. and Primatesta, P. (1999) Health Survey for England. Cardiovascular Disease 1998, *HMSO.*

(16) Bandura, A. (1977) Self-efficacy: Toward a unifying theory of behavioural change. *Psychol. Rev.* 84: 191-215.

(17) Our Healthier Nation – section on 'People and the Communities': a full directory of self-management programmes. (1999) *HMSO.*

(18) The British Liver Trust. Living a Healthy Life with Long-Term Illness (1999) The Board of Trustees, Leland Stanford Junior University.

(19) Barlow, J.H. et al. Self-management literature review. (2000) Psychosocial Research Centre, Coventry University.

(20) Gillies, J., Barry, D., Crane, J., Jones, D., Maclennan, L., Pearce, N., Reid, J. and Troop, L. (1996) A community trial of a written self-management plan for children with asthma. *New Zealand Medical Journal,* 109(1015): 30-33.

(21) Horan, P.P. Yarborough, M.C., Besigel, G. and Carlson, D.R. (1990) Computer assisted self control of diabetes by adolescents. *Diabetes Educator,* 16(3): 205-211.

(22) Skelton, J.R. and Hobbs, F.D. (1999) Concordancing: use of language-based research in medical communication. *The Lancet,* 353: 108-11.

(23) Mandl, K.D., Szolovits, P. and Kohane, I.S. (2001) Public standards of patient control: how to keep electronic records accessible but private. *BMJ,* 322: 283-7.

(24) Piresi, A. (2000) How health literacy prevents equal access to care. *The Lancet,* 356: 1828-12

(25) Kalichman, S.C., Benotsch, E., Suarez, T., Catz, S., Muler, S. and Rampa, D. (2000) Health literacy and health-related knowledge among persons living with HIV AIDS. *Am. J. Prev Med.,* 18: 325-331.

(26) Morrison, R.S., Olsen E., Mertz, K.R. and Meier, D.E. (1995) The inaccessibility of Advance Directives on transfer from ambulatory to acute settings. *JAMA,* 274: 478-82.

(27) Emanuel, L.L. and Emanuel, E.J. (1989) The Medical Directive: a new comprehensive advance care document. *JAMA,* 261: 3288-93.

(28) Emanuel, L.L., Barry, M.J., Stoeckle, J.D., Ettelson, L.M. and Emanuel, E.J. (1991) Advance Directives for medical care – a case for greater use. *New Engl. J. Med.,* 324: 889-95.

(29) Levy, M.L., Davis, S.E., McComb, G. and Apuzzo, M.L.J. (1996) Economic, ethical and outcome-based decisions regarding aggressive surgical management in patients with penetrating craniocerebral injury. *J. Health Communication,* 1: 301-8.

(30) Brody, H., Campbell, M.L., Faber-Lengendoen, K. and Ogle, K.S. (1997) Withdrawing intensive life-sustaining treatment – recommendations for compassionate clinical management. *New Engl. J. Med.* 336: 652-7

(31) Hanson, L.C., Tulsky, J.A. and Danis, M. (1997) Can clinical interventions change care at the end of life? *Ann. Intern. Med.* 126: 381-8.

(32) Smith, A.McC. (2001) Obtaining consent for examination and treatment. *BMJ,* 322: 810-11.

Section 4

The New Medical Paradigm

4.1 21st century patients – resourceful with responsibilities

The 21st century requires not simply another reorganisation but a transformation of the way in which medicine is practised and health-care delivered – a transformation of the health professions, healthcare organisations, and patients. Furthermore, it would not be appropriate to polarise patients and clinicians even further because, although each needs to change, perhaps the most important change necessary is a shift away from the assumption that only the clinician is competent and must bear responsibility for decision making and care organisation. The new paradigm is one in which responsibility and control are shared at a level to be negotiated with each patient. In this final section of the book, the shape of 21st century healthcare is described with respect to:

- patients;
- clinicians;
- organisations.

Finally, a move to shared decision-making is promoted.

4.1 21st century patients – resourceful with responsibilities
4.2 21st century healthcare organisations – patient-centred organisations
4.3 The 21st century clinician – the complementary clinician
4.4 Shared decision-making and patient-centred care

4.1.1 Resources and responsibility

Patients have been given explicit statements of their rights, such as the Human Rights legislation in the year 2000. Rights are expressed both in general terms and in detail, as individual problems have necessitated clarification of patients' rights in particular circumstances. For example, following the discovery that hospitals had received expenses for passing thymus tissue to pharmaceutical companies, the Secretary of State, Alan Milburn, said that 'above all for trust to thrive there has to be informed consent. Not a tick-in-the box consent régime but consent that is based on discussion and dialogue, for consent is actively sought and positively given.' In this book it has been argued that patients also have rights to resources that would allow them to manage their care to a much greater degree than is possible at present. With rights, however, come responsibilities.

4.1.2 Pre-consultation prep and post-consultation homework

Not all patients will wish to avail themselves of the responsibilities and resources that have been described. However, the fundamental contract between patient and clinician in the 21st century should start with the assumption that the patient is competent and responsible, providing they are given the resources to exercise that responsibility. There is a need to recognise that some patients would want to ask the clinician to take responsibility for, among other things, managing their records, arranging all aspects of their care, and taking the lead in decision-making. However, many patients would like to be more involved and to take more responsibility themselves. For those patients who wish to use the resources there will, however, be expectations: they will be expected to prepare for the consultation and, if necessary, do homework after it.

4.1.2.1 Pre-consultation prep

The average consultation in primary care is eight minutes; in secondary hospital care, it is somewhat longer, but in both settings the time is inadequate for complex decision-making. Even though clinicians try to set aside time for longer consultations when they know difficult decisions have to be made, it is often impossible for all relevant issues to be discussed in this period of time. This is particularly so if the patient does not understand the basic language and concepts, because not everyone is well informed about their body, or the process of care.

The resourceful patient would therefore be expected to prepare for the consultation by reading material available on the Web and by ensuring that all the terms, concepts and options that may come up during consultation are understood. The preparation that the patients need depends upon the complexity of the decision they face and the level of understanding they have of health and disease, and basic biology. Using World Wide Web technology, it is relatively simple to ask patients what newspaper they read as a measure of general reading level, and questions about medical terms and concepts to appraise their level of biomedical literacy. On the basis of this appraisal, patients could be offered material to prepare them for the consultation. This could range from videos of patients talking about the decision, and how they had come to make it, to an overview of the authorities, good and bad, right through to the original scientific papers on which medical practice is currently based. Telephone coaching could also be offered. The World Wide Web allows the reader to access detailed information easily and quickly, and in the UK it has been decided that although <u>NHS Direct Online</u> will be offered as the first point of access for patients, all patients will be eligible to access the <u>National electronic Library for Health</u>, prepared primarily for professionals, if they want to know more.

Patients, of course, already have access to the World Wide Web. The difference is that in the context of a health service that expects and supports resourcefulness, the resourceful patient would be using the same information as the clinician. It might be necessary for patients to check that they had understood all the options by testing themselves with standardised questions, so that they could spend more time during the consultation on areas which were still unclear, or perhaps access different ways of explaining it before the start of the consultation. This may sound ambitious, but it does not take months and years of preparation to understand medical documents, or concepts such as the function of the gall bladder or levels of cholesterol.

Furthermore, a systematic review of 22 studies of interactive computerised patient education came to the conclusion that, when used to complement clinical encounters, these techniques improved both the process and outcome of care. Interestingly, they also concluded that 'patients seemed more willing to confide in computers than in human interviewers, possibly because the computers were perceived as non-judgmental.' [1]

Helping people prepare the questions they want to have answered will make life better for clinicians and patients but the limits of the consultation, even with good preparation, should not be underestimated, and post-consultation homework may be required.

4.1.2.2 Post-consultation homework

There is good evidence that, not surprisingly, patients and carers cannot remember everything that is discussed during the consultation. Some clinicians already use cassette recorders to provide the patient and their family with a taped record of the consultation, and this practice is recommended in the guides to improve cancer services in the UK. With new generation palm-tops, this will be easy to do routinely. The patient could be asked to do further work at home before reaching a decision, either to ponder in greater depth on the options considered in the pre-consultation preparation and covered in the consultation, or to think about a new option raised during the consultation. To help with this, the patient could be given written information (on paper or on the Web), a recording of the consultation, and details of a telephone or e-mail decision support service.

4.1.3 The e-consultation

The <u>electronically enhanced consultation</u>, either a face-to-face consultation with prep and homework or an <u>e-mail consultation</u>, described in the Vignette at the end of this book, will allow better decision-making if patients are given resources to accept their responsibilities.

4.1.4 The resourceful patient is nothing new

It has been customary to describe patients as 'highly dependent' if they have been receiving domiciliary care for an hour or two, seven days a week. However, such patients are still without care support for up to 22 hours a day. The resources these people have are limited and largely personal – courage, hope, and a sense of humour. A large independent income also helps, but few have that. However, even those without financial wealth cope remarkably well; with the resources described in this book, patients could cope even better over a wider range of issues than self-care. The resources that patients have called on in the past, resilience and courage, can now be complemented by a range of other resources, perhaps the most important of which is research evidence. The following testimony of one patient demonstrates the importance of this, when he asked (and answered) the question, 'How should I interpret differences of opinion among my medical advisers?' [2]

> In the early 1990s, I broke my ankle while on holiday in the USA. The orthopaedic surgeon I saw there put my leg in a temporary splint. He said that, after the soft-tissue swelling had subsided, the lower leg would be put in a plaster cast for six weeks. At the fracture clinic in my home-town a couple of days later, the orthopaedic surgeon dismissed his American colleague's prescription. Putting the leg in plaster was wholly inappropriate. What was I to make of these differences of opinion? My request for references to good review articles on the natural history and management of fractured fibula was ignored.

The patient's approach is to find a systematic review of the research evidence, and then ask the questions:

Am I sufficiently different from the people included in the review that the evidence can be dismissed confidently as irrelevant to me?

Are the interventions available to me so sufficiently different from those in the review that the evidence can be dismissed confidently as irrelevant to me?

Are the outcomes relevant to me sufficiently different from those in the review that the evidence can be dismissed confidently as irrelevant to me?

He addresses the difficult issue of how one should react to health professionals who shun evidence from systematic reviews of research, and concludes by answering his original question.

Next time I break my ankle I hope that I and my professional advisors will be able to consider the results of systematic reviews of controlled trials comparing lower-leg plastering with strapping for fractured fibula, paying attention to outcomes that are likely to be important to me. Often, the information I would value will not be available, but that is not a reason for ignoring any information that is available. Furthermore, if systematic reviews reveal that there is inadequate evidence to support a clear choice between treatment alternatives, I want to be offered the opportunity to participate in randomised comparisons of the alternative approaches.

Some people might refer to this process as evidence-based patient choice. Whatever it is called, it is motivated in my case not by some unthinking allegiance to a new fad, but by naked self-interest, informed by my professional work over the past three decades.

I have referred to examples of patients who have suffered and died unnecessarily because clinicians have ignored existing research evidence. It is undoubtedly the case that a great deal remains to be done to help all clinicians access reliable, up-to-date information from research, but the practicability of using available evidence in day-to-day clinical practice has been demonstrated.

People who imply that I and other patients should be wary of adopting this approach to the use of research evidence need to show me that, on balance, our approach is less likely than theirs to result in our receiving good healthcare. I shall certainly require something more substantial from them than polemical defences of the status quo – and I shall try to avoid ending up receiving care from any of them who are clinicians.

Although this patient was exceptionally well informed for the year 2000, this level of confidence and competence may be common by 2020.

4.1.5 *Giving patients resources and responsibility for self-management*

Throughout this book we have focused on decision-making and decision-taking but once the decision has been made to institute treatment, patients can be given resources and responsibility for looking after themselves, seeking help only when problems arise. This has long been the case with chronic diseases such as diabetes or asthma but recent evidence demonstrates that the patient can take charge of recurrent episodes of illness.

A study reported in 2001 demonstrated that young women were able to control recurrent attacks of upper urinary tract infection. [3] The research team showed patients how to obtain a clean urine specimen and send the specimen to the laboratory. Patients were also given antibiotics to take if symptoms of urinary tract infection developed. Thus, women in the study who diagnosed that they had a urinary tract infection as a result of the development of symptoms, collected a urine sample and started a course of antibiotics. More than 90 percent of the proven episodes if urinary tract infection were cured without important adverse effects and without the involvement of a clinician, and nearly all of the women who were asked reported that they were confident about managing future urinary tract infections in this way.

4.2 21st century healthcare organisations – patient-centred organisations

Healthcare organisations can help patients become more resourceful by:

- giving patients resources;

- involving patients in the design and running of the service;

- developing systems that assume the patient is resourceful and delivering resources where and when they are needed;

- measuring and acting on the experience of patients;

- helping clinicians become more supportive.

The enquiry into the events at Bristol Royal Infirmary led to a number of principles being proposed to increase public and patient empowerment. These principles, as set out in the Kennedy Report, are reproduced below.

- Patients and the public are entitled to be involved wherever decisions are taken about care in the NHS.

- The involvement of patients and the public must be embedded in the structures of the NHS and permeate all aspects of healthcare.

- The public and patients should have access to relevant information.

- Healthcare professionals must be partners in the process of involving the public and patients.

- There must be honesty about the scope of the public's and patients' involvement, since some decisions cannot be made by the public.

- There must be transparency and openness in the procedures for involving the public and patients.

- The mechanisms for involvement should be evaluated for their effectiveness.

- The public and patients should have access to training and funding to allow them to participate fully.

- The public should be represented by a wide range of individuals and groups and not by particular 'patient groups'.

In 2001, the Department of Health published a Discussion Document on 'Involving the Patients and Public in Healthcare.' A listening exercise was organised and more than a thousand people attended meetings and commented on the proposals. As a result, the Department published a *Response to the Listening Exercise,* which described changes to the initial proposals, and the Secretary of State endorsed these proposals when outlining his Department's response to the Bristol Report with initiatives such as:

- a Patient Advocacy and Liaison Service (PALS) for providing on the spot help for patients within primary care and hospital trusts;

- a Patient Forum for monitoring and reviewing services, and influencing and informing management decisions, in each primary care and hospital trust.

These organisations will be co-ordinated regionally and given national leadership by a Commission for Patient and Public Involvement in Health, which will monitor and improve all these activities, with its authority based on the statutory duty, from the _Health and Social Care Act_, to consult and involve the public.

The private sector has always asserted that it is more sensitive to the needs of patients, and although this has focused on providing faster access and a better environment, they are now focusing on the provision of information. The homepage of _BUPA_, the largest private health service in the UK, now says that 'Informed patients recover faster' because 'patients who understand what is going on can experience less anxiety, less stress, and recover more quickly.' _PPP Healthcare_ provides a service called <u>Health at Hand</u> which 'is ready for your call at any time of the day or night' so that members 'can get easy access to the best health related information.'

4.2.1 Giving resources to patients

The NHS is committed to giving patients:

- electronic patient records to record episodes of care, and
- electronic health records for their lifelong record of health and healthcare.

In addition, healthcare organisations can ensure that:

- their principles and systems are described on a clearly written Web site that conforms to the <u>Bobby</u> principles for disabled access;
- their care pathways are equally open to patients and clinicians;
- information is easily available about local services, and ways in which they may vary from nationally agreed guidelines;
- contracts between clinicians and patients are clear and unambiguous;
- patients are provided with high quality decision aids. A review of the evidence about decision aids shows that they are of benefit to hospitals and healthcare organisations because they have the effects shown in Table 12. [4]

However, patients should not only be seen as passive recipients of resources – they can be actively involved in the planning and management of care.

Table 1: Do decision aids work?
Evaluation studies from a Cochrane systematic overview

Decision aids improve decision-making by:

- reducing the proportion of patients who are uncertain about what to choose;

- increasing patients' knowledge of the problem, options and outcomes;

- creating realistic personal expectation (perceived probabilities) of outcomes;

- improving the agreement between choices and a patients' values;

- reducing some elements of decisional conflict (feeling uncertain, uninformed, unclear about values, and unsupported in decision-making);

- increasing participation in decision-making without adversely affecting anxiety

---

4.2.2 Involving patients for better care

Patients or their representatives can be involved:

- on the Board of healthcare organisations;

- on patient participation groups working with clinicians to improve services;

- in the design of new facilities;

- in research projects.

The involvement of patients in research is perhaps the most radical of these moves. It has been customary for research to be governed by ethics committees to ensure that patients are protected from poorly designed or harmful research projects. Interestingly, although research ethics is of great importance, there is some evidence that patients are safer and better cared for when they are involved in a research project, and therefore that ethical concern should focus not only on the researcher who wishes to test a hypothesis but also on the clinician or service manager who wishes to introduce new treatments or services. Hitherto, the latter groups had no controls at all placed on their behaviour when they wished to introduce a new treatment or service.

In the 1990s, patients began to be involved in the design and execution of research, not only to make the research more acceptable but to improve the relevance and usefulness of the research. The Cochrane Collaboration has made the involvement of patients central to its work since its inception, because the involvement of patients and carers ensures that the right questions are asked and the right conclusions are drawn from data. The Director of the UK Cochrane Centre has illustrated the benefits of this approach by pointing out that if women had been involved in the design of breast cancer treatment trials much earlier, the problem of radiation injury to the upper arm would have been identified much earlier because clinicians focused principally on cancer mortality as their outcome measure.

Guidelines were initially written by clinicians for clinicians but the North of England Evidence-based Guideline Development Project explained four different ways of involving consumers, as set out below.

The four methods explored were:

- incorporating individual patients in guideline development groups;
- a 'one off' meeting with patients;
- a series of workshops with patients;
- incorporating a consumer advocate in guideline development groups.

The key messages were:

- consumers should be involved in all the stages of guideline development to ensure their views are heard. Consumers (like all guideline development group members) need support to be able to understand the detail of the science behind the issues they will hear about and contribute to the discussion;
- having explored four different methods of involving consumers, none was ideal and, even if optimised, each alone would be likely to remain limited;
- given the greater degree of discussion within a 'one off' group of patients than by the sole patients within the guideline groups, it seems reasonable to at least offer consumers within guideline

groups the option of being one of a pair;

• it is feasible to support consumers to understand the technical elements of guideline development. (5)

The message is clear. Patients should, and can, be involved in guideline development and the <u>National Institute for Clinical Excellence</u> does this.

4.2.3 Developing systems that deliver resources when and where they are needed

A system is a set of activities with a common set of objectives. Healthcare organisations deliver systems of care to diagnose and treat patients. There must also be systems that provide resources for patients when and where they are needed.

The classic example is the informed consent form, usually given as a paper document to a patient before an operation or procedure. However, digital television will soon be at every patient's bedside, paradoxically giving the patients better access to screens than clinicians. As well as letting the patient watch diverting films and shows, these screens could also be used to offer the patient about to undergo a procedure or operation:

• background information about the procedure and what will happen;

• information about the probabilities of benefit and harm, including the ability to deliver this information to people of different reading age;

• videos of the experience of other individual patients who have undergone the same procedure or operation, through the DIPEX database.

These resources can also reduce medical error, but when medical error occurs, it is important for the health service to be open and honest. The Secretary of State set out seven pledges for quality improvement in September 2001.

4.2.4 Measuring and acting on the patient's experience of care

The resourceful patient not only needs resources but acts as a resource for the intelligent clinician or manager. Patient satisfaction is largely determined by expectation: patients can be satisfied with very poor quality care if expectations are low. Because of the weakness of patient satisfaction as a measure of service quality, important though it is, the <u>Picker Institute</u>, founded in the US and now active in Europe, developed systematic methods for measuring patients experience of the care they received. The Picker survey asks questions not only about the hospital environment but also about communication and clinical decision-making (Box 1).

Examples of questions on the Picker Institute Patient Survey

G3   Beforehand did a member of staff explain the risks and benefits of the operation or procedure in a way you could understand?

G4   Beforehand did a member of staff answer your questions about the operation or procedure in a way you could understand?

H5   Did a doctor explain the purpose of the medicines you were to take at home in a way you could understand?

For example, rather than asking people if they were satisfied with the amount of information given, they were asked to recollect what information had been given. If the patient could not recollect any information, that fact is important to the healthcare organisation, whether or not the clinician thought that the information had been transmitted, and whether or not the patient was satisfied with the amount of information received. The measurement of the experience provides a direct measure of service quality and patients are resources of great value to those who provide or pay for healthcare.

4.2.5 Screening programmes now assume that people are resourceful

The word 'screen' originally meant a sieve – something used for sifting coal or grain, but in the last hundred years the meaning of the word has changed, and it now signifies something that is solid and impervious, a screen in a cinema or the folded screen in the corner of a room, over which, in a stage farce, clothing can be tantalisingly draped while the naked person is kept perfectly hidden. In medical screening, the original meaning of the word is much more appropriate, for two reasons:

- no screening programme is able to detect all the cases of disease in a population, and

- every screening programme classifies some people with a positive diagnosis when they do not have the disease.

This is analogous to a sieve used for sifting grain. The objective of this sieve is to let through dust, small stones and chaff whilst retaining the grain, but in practice:

- some grain falls through the holes in the sieve, and

- some stones and chaff are retained in the sieve.

Of course it is possible to construct the perfect sieve, but

- if the holes are made so small that not a single drop of grain will fall through, lots of dust, dirt and chaff will be retained inside the sieve;

- if the holes are made big enough for every bit of dust, dirt and chaff to fall out of the sieve, lots of grain will drop through to the ground.

Every screening programme, therefore, has

- false positives: people who are told they have the disease but who do not actually have it, and

- false negatives: people for whom the screening test is negative but who do actually have the disease.

It is impossible to have a screening programme with no false negatives and no false positives.

4.2.5.1 Disillusionment with screening

There was great confidence in screening when medical hubris was at its height. It seemed obvious that to find disease early would result in better outcomes, but this is not always true. There are many reasons for this. One reason is that some cancers may have spread at a very early stage, which makes even early detection through screening ineffective in increasing the probability of cure. Screening created an image of 100% perfection, but the systematic measurement of error demonstrated by the quality assurance systems developed for screening programmes has shown that this is not the case, leading to disillusionment with screening. However, this disillusionment is not so much with the screening process itself, because people offered screening can very quickly appreciate the fact that screening programme cannot be 100% sensitive and specific. But what they feel is that they have been misled.

4.2.5.2 The drive to maximise coverage

Before health care planners took the views of patients and the public seriously, they took a utilitarian and businesslike approach to screening. They saw screening as offering potential benefits for some of the individuals screened, and for the population as a whole. Healthcare planners sought to encourage people to attend for screening, and to motivate healthcare professionals to increase their enthusiasm to persuade people to attend for screening. General practitioners, for example, were paid depending upon the proportion of their population that had had a cervical smear, leading one woman to complain that 'I have had four letters asking me to go for cervical screening. When will they ever learn that I do not want to go?' It is certainly appropriate to point out the potential benefits of screening to people, but what screening programmes did not point out, until recently, were the inherent problems in screening, in that:

- all screening programmes do harm to some people;
- some of the people who are harmed do not have the disease for which they are screened.

In clinical practice clinicians offer treatment, and patients know that there is a probability of harm; not perhaps as well as they should know, but the contract between clinician and patient is still clear. In screening, however, some of the people screened will have a false positive result, and they will be harmed as a result of the investigations that are offered to them, from which they stand no possibility of gaining benefit because they do not have the disease. For example, in screening for colorectal cancer, the initial screening test for blood in the faeces is simple and harmless. However, those who test positive have a colonoscopy, a procedure which is not without risk, resulting as it can in perforation of the colon, which can lead to peritonitis, and even to death. This series of events could occur in some people who do not have the disease, and for this reason screening, more than any service, needs to treat all those who undergo it as intelligent adults.

The national breast and cervical screening programmes were the first to identify the need to:

- emphasise that screening did not detect all cancers;

- emphasise that screening was potentially harmful;

- offer informed choice.

In a research project designed to help the national breast cancer screening programme provide clear information, it was proposed that all women be offered clear and accurate information about the risks and limitations of screening.

Table 13: Advantages and disadvantages of screening
Potential benefits and difficulties of breast screening
• Most breast cancers are found at an early stage when there is a good chance of a successful recovery.
• Around half the cancers found at screening are still small enough to allow breast saving surgery.
• Breast screening is estimated to save about 1,250 lives per year in the UK.
• Breast screening reduces the risk of dying from breast cancer in the women who attend.
• Some women will be recalled for rurther investigations because of uncertainties over their mammogram. Following further tests, many of these will prove not to have cancer. Being recalled can cause unnecessary worry.
• Some breast cancers present will be missed by screening.
• Not all breast cancers found at screening can be cured.
• Many women find mammography painful albeit for a brief period of time.

This approach has been taken in other screening programmes. Antenatal screening is obviously an area in which open and complete information is absolutely essential, partly because one of the outcomes in antenatal screening is abortion. It is therefore essential to tell women about the possible consequences of a blood test before that test is taken.

The <u>National Screening Committee</u> in the United Kingdom has proposed that screening be renamed as 'risk reduction' to try to emphasise the fact that it is not 100% sensitive or specific. The committee also introduced the concept of 'informed choice' for all screening programmes and argued that if health care professionals are to be paid, this should not be based on the proportion of the population that has been persuaded to have a test but on the proportion of the population that feels that it has been empowered to make an informed choice. The National Screening Committee organised a workshop on informed choice in screening which examined this concept, and ways in which it could be introduced in different types of screening programmes. The workshop recognised that there was a conflict between giving information to encourage uptake and giving information which might lead to the person invited to be screened not accepting the offer, which could reduce both the uptake and cost effectiveness of screening programmes. In a paper addressing the ethics of informed choice, the author emphasised the need to respect the principle of autonomy, particularly in screening programmes. The way to do this was by encouraging a new style of consultation in which the consideration of choice was regarded as its most important function, whatever the choice made at the end of that consultation. [6]

4.2.5.3 Where screening leads, other services will follow

Because screening services deal with healthy people, and can cause harm to them, the moral responsibility of those involved in the management and delivery of screening is generally considered to be greater than that of clinical practice. However, many of the principles that have been developed in the screening programme are equally relevant to clinical practice, and there appears to be no qualitative difference between the two types of health service. As a result, there is no good reason why the principles and practices developed in screening should not be applied throughout all of healthcare.

4.2.5.4 Making offers to punters

'Well, Dr Gray, we have had a long discussion about whether we should call people patients or clients. "Patients" is not a very good word for people invited for screening but neither is "clients". The best thing would be to call them "punters" because, let's face it, Dr Gray, they are taking a chance every time they walk into the service.'

This doctor's remark, intended to be flippant, made at a meeting considering what people offered screening should be called, was received with great enthusiasm by professional colleagues because the word 'punter', in the United Kingdom at least, is used to describe someone who is taking a gamble. The person who is the punter needs to know not simply about whether there is evidence about the effectiveness of cervical screening but about the relevance of cervical screening to them as an individual. The punter's age is of significance and in a paper in the *Journal of the American Medical Association,* the changing relevance of the age factor in screening for cervical, breast and colorectal cancer was considered. Screening has a probability of benefit for each individual and a probability of harm, and depending upon the individual's age, and certain other health factors, the probability of benefit and the probability of harm vary. The authors of the paper present two different case studies outlined below.

> *Case I. Mrs A is a 75-year-old white woman with diabetes, severe dementia, and functional dependency in all activities of daily living. She lives with her daughter and has no prior history of any cancer screening tests.*

> *Case 2. Miss B is an 80-year-old white woman who is widowed, living with her sister. She has no comorbid conditions, walks 3 miles a day, and cooks and cleans for her older sister. She has no prior history of any cancer screening tests.*

Having presented a lot of data about the probability of dying, the probability of benefit and the probability of harm, the authors relate this method to the two cases.

'Mrs A has avoided physicians all her life and does not like undergoing tests'. On the other hand, 'Miss B reveals that she worries about her health and wants to have a mammogram, a pap smear and a faecal occult blood test for colonic cancer'. The decision is therefore to recommend that Mrs A should not be given a screening test but that Miss B should be given a screening test even if her probability of benefit is relatively low. [7] In an accompanying editorial [8] the author, who is an influential physician, not only reflects on the article but also tells how he had just spent time with his 80-year-old mother who had asked him to write down all the relevant information about the treatment of narrowing of the carotid arteries, which can include radical surgery. Having reflected on his experience in the article, the author of the editorial states that he 'cannot imagine trying to communicate all these ideas to my mother, or any other patient, in a fifteen minute visit. Because screening has been so effectively promoted as a uniform good, these ideas may be seen as heretical to most.' He does, however, emphasise that educational efforts formerly focused on persuading people to be screened, have had to focus on the trade-offs, and although screening is beneficial for populations, it is for many patients what the Americans call 'a close call'.

4.2.6 21st century healthcare industries – advertising medicines

In giving patients full information about their medicines, pharmaceutical companies are required to produce descriptions of the drugs they produce and to make this information available to patients. This is usually done by printing information on a small sheet of paper, in small or very small type, necessarily so because the printing of the information in the type size and spacing of this book produces a sheet of paper that would require a pillbox to be much larger than it is at present. The Association of British Pharmaceutical Industries, the ABPI, is keen to give patients full access to information and has a working party on the informed patient which is promoting better and fuller information for patients.

If medicines are legal, as they are, and if patients are intelligent, as they are, the ban on advertising medicines is difficult to sustain. In the United States medicines can be advertised and the distinction between advertising and informing, or between promotion and information, which may be difficult to discern in Europe, is now clearly different in America, where drugs can be advertised to patients, with the advertisers using the same powerful overt and covert messages as they use for other products.

In Europe there is opposition to the advertising of medicines, in part because it is thought that this will increase the demand for medicines. Most governments are keen for the pharmaceutical industry to provide high quality information to the patient once the decision to prescribe has been made, but wish to shield the patient from intensive advertising before the decision is made as to whether or not to prescribe medicine, or the decision is made as to which particular medicine should be chosen.

The strict adherence of the pharmaceutical industry to these guidelines is praiseworthy but their usefulness was called into question by the dramatic sales figures for Viagra, which was not provided by the NHS or most other healthcare providers in Europe, but which was obtained in large amounts by ageing males. There was no need for the drug company to advertise – the Internet did the job, and more patients will gain the information about their medicines from drug companies on the Web – and it is right that they should do so – once the decision has been made about which medicine they should have.

Drug companies are now doing even more – for example, Pfizer, in an advertisement in *The British Medical Journal,* now advertises to inform the journal's readers (doctors) that their publication, *Your Heart* is 'mailed directly to patients' homes; *Your Heart* is a unique educational programme for patients starting treatment with Istin™, Cardura™, Lipitor™. This includes 'a workbook, personal action plan, monthly fact sheets and newsletters to encourage patient responsibility.'

The Association of the British Pharmaceutical Industry commissioned a report on *The Expert Patient* to inform their project called 'The Informed Patient Initiative', and the report, which proposed a new 'Patients' Code', concluded that:

> *The most important thing is to recognise that different patients have different needs – and that the same patients may have different needs at different times in their lives.*
>
> *There is no one right way. Some patients will want to establish a 'sharing partnership' with their doctors in which they weigh up the options and decide together what to do for the best. Others may feel this is inappropriate if the doctor is under pressure to rein in prescribing costs, arguing that a partnership involves sharing in equal measure, and that the doctor-patient relationship is by definition unequal. Some will continue to opt for the paternalistic model. Each of these models had a valid place in the overall scheme of things. But the development of the expert patient is an unstoppable trend.*

Another new type of service is called LinkMedica.which is of interest not only because it is funded by a drug company, AstraZeneca, but also because it offers a completely new way of helping doctors and patients work together to achieve better control of asthma. The online service provided through LinkMedica would allow a patient with asthma to:

● monitor their asthma over the Internet or by telephone daily;

● obtain immediate feedback on how she is managing her asthma;

● share the daily information with her doctor or nurse;

● obtain current pollen and pollution counts for the part of the country in which they live.

All of it is backed by a knowledge centre, which clearly distinguishes between 'evidence-based content' and 'news', with the evidence-based content being written reports of findings from 'the best available clinical research', and these are made equally open to health professionals and patients.

The service offers an electronic asthma diary, which allows the patient to record her symptoms andcertain physiological signs. When this information is fed to the Asthma Management Centre, the patient receives electronically, a clear signal, either green, yellow, orange or red, about the actions he needs to take to avoid an acute episode, which often results in hospitalisation. The site is justified by a piece of evidence-based content, namely a review of 22 clinical trials which compared people who were treated for asthma in the usual manner with those who had learned self-management techniques, and this review showed that structured self-management reduced hospital admissions and time off from work or school. LinkMedica demonstrates, however, that self-management can be supported through the Internet, allowing new patterns of care to evolve.

4.2.7 Helping clinicians become supportive

One of the most important functions the healthcare organisation can undertake is to support those clinicians who deliver care directly to patients, and who will have to evolve quickly and dramatically to adapt to resourceful patients.

4.3 The 21st century clinician – the complementary clinician

> 'The key question to ask is what is the function of the human being in the digital age?'
>
> Bill Gates

Bill Gates' question was posed for people who manage service industries such as banks or travel agents, but it is equally relevant for those who run health services and for clinicians themselves. The question could also be posed by asking, 'what is the function of the clinician in the consumer age?' but these two questions are inter-related because the Internet gives consumers new and unprecedented powers, and consumerism gives the patient the confidence to expect a service that meets their individual needs. The clinician in the 21st century therefore has to complement the skills and resources of each patient and be different things to different patients, supporting decision-making for the patient who wants to make all the decisions herself but taking decisions when the patient has made it clear that she wants the clinician to take the final decision and organise care appropriately. The clinician of the 21st century will also have to be:

- a good mechanic, and

- a sensitive human being.

4.3.1 The clinician must be a master mechanic

The statement that 'no patient should be treated by a below average clinician' epitomises a problem for both clinician and patient. Below average sounds unacceptable but being below average is for a proportion of clinicians or any other group, inevitable and inescapable, and 50% of clinicians will always be 'below average'. There is, however, increasing concern among patients about below average services, which may be confused with low levels of quality. The latter are unacceptable, the former are inevitable, but patients are, understandably, less tolerant of errors in healthcare and below average clinical practice.

Two official reports of medical errors in the United States and the United Kingdom [9,10] revealed just how common such errors are. Furthermore, it is clear that some of these errors are not preventable but are inherent in the process of complex decision-making and the delivery of technologically sophisticated healthcare. However, this is not an argument for complacency, and errors can and must be reduced in both incidence and severity. Similarly, all clinicians must be helped to become better at practising their calling, and the profession as a whole is keen to do this, although it is sometimes felt that both the public and politicians overlook the barriers that clinicians have to face and overcome if they are to deliver acceptable, or excellent, quality care. To improve mutual understanding, the <u>General Medical Council</u>, the medical profession's ruling body, has set up a Patient Reference Group to allow patients a greater say in the evolution of the profession.

One barrier is the fact that the clinician is faced with a huge amount of knowledge which changes and increases remorselessly. A study of general practitioners showed that by the end of 1998, each had been sent 22 kg of guidelines; it is estimated that to keep up with developments in medicine as a general practitioner or physician, it would be necessary to read twenty scientific papers every day. The only option for the 21st century physician is to recognise the truth of a proposition by Dr David Pencheon, cited in the *British Medical Journal*, that the three most important words for the clinician of the future are 'I don't know.' Instead of using the clinician as a repository of the knowledge, the clinician should be a knowledge manager, that is someone who can:

- ask the right question and find the best answer;

- help the patient interpret the knowledge he has been given or has found for himself.

To be a knowledge manager, the clinician has to have easy access to best current knowledge, and this is sadly lacking at the moment. The young mechanic at a Ford garage is provided with the knowledge he needs, available within seconds. If something needs attention on a Boeing aircraft engine, every mechanic who requires it will be given the knowledge to repair it that same day. In the middle of the night the young clinician on a hospital ward may have no access to the Internet or any other easily accessible source of best current knowledge. Equally, if knowledge has to be distributed to increase the safety of healthcare, it can take months or years to arrive, or may never arrive in the form most likely to be helpful. This makes the job of the clinician even more difficult because the clinician has to be much more than a mechanic: she has to complement the resources of the patient.

4.3.1.1 *Master mechanics need decent workshops*

Clinicians need access to best current knowledge, whenever and wherever they see patients. The National electronic Library for Health now offers easy access but only if clinicians can get their hands on a keyboard and their eyes on a screen, and for many clinicians, this is impossible. The NHS Information Authority is now taking steps to get the infrastructure in place, in partnership with the big players in the computer industry such as Cisco, Oracle, and Microsoft, but massive changes are needed to transform health services, and the Department of Health has set up a Modernisation Agency to accelerate change. Highly trained mechanics cannot do their job if they are given no more than a hammer.

4.3.2 *Complementing the patient's resources*

In the 20th century, the clinician's task was determined by a number of variables such as:

- the state of knowledge about a health problem;

- the health service;

- resources available;

- the patient's diagnosis and clinical condition;

- the clinician's training and expertise.

All these are still relevant to 21st century clinical practice, but the focus in the 21st century, and the clinician's approach to a patient, are now influenced by other factors, notably:

- the value patients attribute to health improvement and the adverse effects that might occur as a result of treatment;

- the resources that the patient has available to participate in decision-making about management and care, for example whether or not the patient has access to the World Wide Web;

- the style of decision-making desired by the patient;

- the experience and skill of the patient in decision-making and care management;

- the clinician's skill in, and attitude towards, shared decision-making.

Attitudes influence professional behaviour, and not all professionals are equally committed to making resources available to patients. Pregnant women, one expects, would be a group that clinicians would want to see well informed because they are healthy people being helped on a journey which is usually safe, with a pleasant outcome. Excellent information is available for pregnant women, in the form of leaflets based on best current knowledge, specifically designed to promote informed choice by the Midwives Information and Resource Service. A study of professional reactions to the leaflets found that although midwives thought them helpful, the clinicians who carried out the ultrasound examination were concerned that the message was too negative and would create unnecessary anxiety. Furthermore, they feared that the provision of too much information might have an adverse affect on the relationship between clinician and patient. [11] The changes taking place within professions are not always welcome, and the President of the General Medical Council, Sir Donald Irvine, was frequently criticised for the introduction of changes essential for the continuing independence of the medical profession.

Hostile attitudes to change are becoming less common, partly because clinicians now know that for medico-legal reasons they must offer all the information about the risks and limitations of the services they provide. They are also in decline because of a genuine commitment to patient centred consultations, which focus on high quality communication and a sense of partnership, as well as the traditional function of the consultation, as a means of finding and solving problems.

4.3.2.1 Patient preferences for consulting style

It is important to remember that not all patients want the same style of consultation. Furthermore, the evidence is that clinicians, not surprisingly, do not always identify the style of decision making that patients want. In one study of women with breast cancer, showing a range of preferences for different types of decision making:

- 42% of women achieved their preferred level of control;

- 14.9% of women believed they had been pushed to take more control than they wanted;

- 21% of the women who wanted the most active level of responsibility for decision making – 22% of all women – achieved it.[12]

Direct observation of 1057 consultations in the United States found that only 9.0% of consultations had completely satisfactory communication and decision-making. Even more worryingly, it found that only 1.5% of consultations were deemed to have assessed the level of the patient's understanding,[13] leading the author of an editorial accompanying the article to state that, if the profession is to achieve shared decision making 'we, as physicians, must do a better job of practising what we preach.' [14]

4.3.2.2. The end of 'compliance'

Analogous to the term 'consent' is the term 'compliance' which is used to describe the degree to which the patient conforms with the therapeutic 'régime', another term with connotations of control and power. The term 'compliance' is usually employed when describing the taking of prescribed medication – good compliance means the patient takes the drugs as prescribed, poor compliance means they don't. In an attempt to reframe the relationship, the Royal Pharmaceutical Society of Great Britain, which governs the practice of pharmacists, has proposed the use of the term 'concordance' and has defined this term.

Concordance has also been called partnership in medicine-taking; it has been defined as building a therapeutic alliance. It's a complex recipe, but here are three crucial ingredients:

Concordance includes an explicit agreement between two people – even if the two agree to differ. One person's impression that an agreement has been reached is not enough.

Concordance is based on respect for each other's beliefs. We reject the idea that one group of people (health care professionals) is objective, expert and rational, while another (patients) is subjective, ignorant and irrational. Patients are often experts on their own condition. We all (patients and professionals) need to respect the right of others to think differently – and take strength from embracing the opposing view.

Concordance gives the patient the casting vote. If the patient wants the professional to rake all the decisions, that's fine. But if the patient and prescriber agree to differ, we recognise that the patient's view comes first. Taking medicines is a kind of experiment, which can only take place if the patient wants it to.

Many of the examples in this book describe the inter-action between doctor and patient, but the issues are equally relevant for all clinicians, dentists, nurses, and therapists. Some of these groups, notably nurses, have been quicker to appreciate the need to take the patient's perspective. As these other professions are given more power and more direct responsibility for decision-making and support, these principles and practices will become even more relevant and important.

4.3.3 The clinician as human being

In response to Mr Gates' challenge, the clinician has to focus on the human side of clinical practice in the 21st century. Some of the techniques that clinicians have formerly used unaided can now be supported by computing and the World Wide Web, such as:

- taking a comprehensive and complete history;

- finding best current knowledge;

- choosing the most appropriate tests;

- relating research knowledge and test results to the individual patient.

No clinician is now in a position to know everything or be absolutely sure they are up to date, and why should they be? These are tasks which human beings can do if they super-specialise and spend their life in study. In the 21st century, knowledge management is dramatically facilitated by the World Wide Web and human beings may concentrate on tasks that computers and the Web cannot do.

It is important, however, that clinicians are not complacent about their human powers. Many clinicians, for example, claim that they are able to offer empathy to patients, but interviews demonstrate that some patients have found that Internet chat rooms offer better support than clinicians. The personality of the clinician may give the impression that they either have the empathic sensitivity or that they do not, but what has been revealed is that many physicians are predisposed to provide empathy and support for patients but that their behaviour does not always indicate this. Clinical students are increasingly taught not only to be clear in the consultation but also to give the right leads to patients. For example, interviews with patients and the observations of consultations have allowed guidelines for clinical empathy to be developed (Table 13) and statements that facilitate empathy to be identified and taught (Table 14).[15] Despite this, human sensitivity, if well developed, still offers receptivity far beyond that of the computer.

Table 13: Guidelines for clinical empathy in the cross-cultural setting

Understand your own cultural values and biases.

Develop a familiarity with the cultural values, health beliefs, and illness behaviours of ethnic, cultural, and religious groups served in your practice.

Ask how the patient prefers to be addressed.

Determine the patient's level of fluency in English and arrange for a translator, if needed.

Assure the patient of confidentiality; rumours, jealousy, privacy, and reputation are crucial issues in close-knit traditional communities.

Use a speech rate, tone, and style that promote understanding and show respect for the patient.

Check back frequently to determine patient understanding and acceptance.

Table 14: Words that work: statements that facilitate empathy

Queries

'Would you (or could you) tell me a little more about that?'
'What has this been like for you?'
'Is there anything else?'
'Are you OK with that?'
'Hmmmm...'

Clarification

'Let me see if I have this right.'
'I want to make sure I really understand what you're telling me. I am hearing that ...'
'I don't want us to go further until I'm sure I've got it right.'
'When I'm done, if I've gone astray, I'd appreciate it if you would correct me. OK?'

Responses

'That sounds very difficult.'
'Sounds like ...'
'That's great! I bet you're feeling pretty good about that.'
'I can imagine that this might feel ...'
'Anyone in your situation would feel that way ...'
'I can see that you are ...'

Human sensitivity is particularly important where subtle influences are crucial. When a patient is incompetent, or unconscious, or a minor, his ability to be resourceful is obviously impaired, and special arrangements are in place to ensure good decision-making. When, however, the patient is competent, but is poorer and much older than the clinician, or less well-educated, or of a different race, class or gender, decision-making can be compromised. There is evidence that people who differ from clinicians in these ways have different experiences, often with different outcomes, than patients of the same class, age, race and educational level as the clinician. For example, one study of patients in the US who were elderly, poor and black, found them to have higher rates of feeding through a tube placed through the skin into the stomach – a gastrostomy tube – even though this procedure had a substantial mortality rate of 15.3%.[16] Another study, of patients over 65 with heart disease in Liverpool, found that 'patients from deprived areas may be less confident in dealing with doctors than their more affluent neighbours' and concluded that cultural barriers reduced the probability of elderly poor patients being referred for effective treatment despite 'all but one patient having English as their first language.' [17]

Prejudice, conscious or unconscious, is one explanation for such differences. However, the explanation may be more subtle, with even the least prejudiced clinician having problems with communication. Clinicians need practical advice about the best way to seek consent.

4.3.4 A practical guide to obtaining consent for treatment

The Christmas edition of the *British Medical Journal* is always a joy. Many of the articles are tongue-in-cheek, but the court jester style allows things to be said which never could be said in the serious editions of the journal on the other fifty weeks of the year (the bumper Christmas edition covers two weeks).

In a paper in the Christmas 2001 edition, three of the leaders of the evidence-based medicine initiative gave 'a practical guide to informed consent to treatment'.

Interactive, personalised approach to informed consent:

'Good morning, Mrs Jones. My name is Dr Smith. Please sit down and make yourself comfortable. Your GP has probably explained to you that he has asked me to see you because your breathlessness doesn't seem to be getting any better, and he wondered whether I might be able to suggest ways of helping. I hope I will be able to do so, but this may well mean seeing you on several occasions over the next few months and working together to find the best treatment for your condition.

'I'm more likely to be able to help if I can get to know more about you and your priorities and preferences. As this is the first time we've met, I thought it might be helpful to mention briefly how I will try to do this. Patients vary in the amount of information that they want to give to and receive from their doctors. Most patients seem to get less information from their doctors than they want, but others would rather not be told some of the things that doctors assume they must want to know. Because you and I don't know each other yet, I'm going to need your help in learning how much information you want about your problem, and about the possible treatment options. I'm going to depend on you to prompt me to give you more information if you think I'm not being

sufficiently forthcoming, or to tell me that you've heard enough if you think I'm overdoing it. You also need to know that I will never lie in response to a straight question from you, and if I don't know the answer I will do my best to find it for you. Does that seem to you to be an acceptable way of proceeding?'[18]

4.3.4 Partnerships between resourceful patients and complementary clinicians

The most important principle for the future is that of partnership.

4.4 Shared decision-making and patient-centred care

Things cannot go on in the same old way. Health care has never been so effective, as measured objectively, or so much criticised and self-criticised, as measured subjectively.

A leader in the *British Medical Journal* [19] by its bold and perceptive editor, Richard Smith asks, 'Why are doctors so unhappy?', and answers this question by saying that there is a 'bogus contract' between doctor and patient and that this bogus contract needs to be replaced by a new contract. Smith's elegant analysis of the bogus contract and his proposal for a new contract is summarised in the box below (Table 15).

The importance of perception cannot be underestimated. Doctors in both the United States and the United Kingdom believe that they have less time for each patient, yet objective measures, described in an article in the *British Medical Journal*, show that time spent with patients is increasing in both countries.[20] This article, entitled 'How should hamsters run?' summarises the impression that doctors have of themselves as being like hamsters in a wheel.

The position is serious but not hopeless. New technologies, such as e-mail consultation as described in the hamster article, offer new opportunities for working in different ways.

Of even greater importance than the need to deliver the old-style consultation in new and slicker ways, however, is the need to redefine the consultation and the practice of medicine. Furthermore, this requires not only a broader definition of the concept of medicine as embodied, for example, in the concept of integrated medicine[21], but also a fundamental realignment of the relationship between clinician and patient, sometimes called 'patient-centred care'.

Table 15: Doctors and patients: redrafting a bogus contract

The bogus contract: the patient's view

- Modern medicine can do remarkable things: it can solve many of my problems.

- You, the doctor, can see inside me and know what's wrong.

- You know everything it's necessary to know.

- You can solve my problems, even my social problems.

- So we give you high status and a good salary.

The bogus contract: the doctor's view

- Modern medicine has limited powers.

- Worse, it's dangerous.

- We can't begin to solve all problems, especially social ones.

- I don't know everything, but I do know how difficult many things are.

- The balance between doing good and harm is very fine.

- I'd better keep quiet about all this so as not to dissapoint my patients and lose my status.

The new contract

Both patients and doctors know:

- Death, sickness and pain are part of life.

- Medicine has limited powers, particularly to solve social problem, and is risky.

- Doctors don't know everything: they need decision making and psychological support.

- We're in this together.

- Patients can't leave problems to doctors.

- Doctors should be open about their limitations.

- Politicians should refrain from extravagant promises and concentrate on reality.

4.4.1 Patient-centred care

Even allowing for the fact the past is often viewed through rose-tinted spectacles, many people talk about an era when they had better relationships with the clinicians who treated them. This was, however, a time in which the patient was clearly subservient to the clinician (Figure 13).

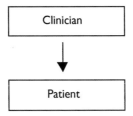

Figure 13

In the past ten years, clinicians and patients have drifted into a more adversarial relationship. Part of the reason for this is that patients have changed and new cohorts of patients who have grown up in an era of consumerism, suspicious of modern science, do not want a return to the subservient relationship. For the 21st century the relationship will evolve to become one of partnership between, on the one hand, healthcare organisations and clinicians and, on the other, patients and their representatives (Figure 14).

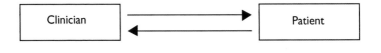

Figure 14

The balance differs from patient to patient and clinician to clinician, and the relationship between each patient and clinician lies on a continuum. In some relationships, at the left-hand of the spectrum (Figure 15), the patient will bear more responsibility; but in all the consultations decision-making will be shared.

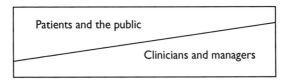

Figure 15

The definition of 'patient-centred care' varies from one culture to another but certain common themes emerge, embodied in five questions published in a paper developed under the sponsorship of the <u>American Academy on Physician and Patient</u>[22]. The five key questions are:

- Who is this patient?

- What does this patient want from the physician and the medical team?

- How does the patient experience this illness?

- What are the patient's ideas about the illness?

- What are the patient's main feelings about the illness?

Although this approach was developed in family practice, it is of relevance and importance to all aspects of health care and clinical practice. Central to the development of patient-centred care is a commitment not only to give high priority to the patient's view of the problem, and the health service with which they are interacting, but also to promote shared decision-making.

4.4.1.1 Better organised patients

This book has focused on the consultation because that is where most crunch decisions are made between the clinician and patient. Outside the consultation the clinician, however, is a member of, and is supported by, a number of organisations and societies, whereas the patient is usually a lone agent supported by an informal network of family and friends. The informal network can, of course, be very powerful; love and concern are strong sources of support, but it is usually poorly informed with few resources. These informal networks are now complemented by well organised 'patients' groups.

The growth of these groups, sometimes called mutual aid societies, has been one of the striking features of healthcare in almost every disease or health problem in the last two decades of the twentieth century. Some are large and well funded, usually because they deal with common problems such as diabetes or heart disease, whereas those which support people with a rare disease, or their carers, depend largely on the resources provided by fellow sufferers, usually supported by the leading doctors who have a special interest in that problem. The smaller organisation may sometimes join a larger umbrella one, such as the <u>Long-Term Medical Conditions Alliance</u> or

<u>Contact a Family</u>, and the <u>Patients' Forum</u> now acts as the one focus for all this activity with its remit being to:

> *promote wider discussion of current health issues among the whole raft of organisations representing patients and carers;*

> *improve arrangements for communication, timely consultation and liaison between the health consumer network and Government, and relevant societies and professional organisations.*

These societies offer the opportunity for institutional shared decision-making to complement individual shared decision-making in the consultation. Leading clinicians are often influential in these societies, many of which also raise money for research, and, increasingly, representatives from the societies are involved by the professions and government in their committees and working groups. In 2001, for example, that venerable institution, the Royal College of Physicians, appointed the Chief Executive of the patients' group <u>Diabetes UK</u> to chair an influential committee. Patients are now not only better informed but also better organised but that offers the medical profession an excellent opportunity for partnership.

4.4.2 *Learning from Bristol*

On 17 January 2002, the Secretary of State for Health, Alan Milburn, presented the government's response to the report of the public inquiry in children's heart surgery at the Bristol Royal Infirmary, known as the Kennedy Report. The Department of Health's response, *Learning from Bristol*, dealt with all of the recommendations made in the Kennedy Report, emphasising that they were going to put patients at the centre of the NHS and 'improve quality, reliability and the range of information which supports decision-making.'

The report calls for a culture of openness and honesty, and makes specific recommendations about the need for patients to be involved in decision-making. The report says patients 'should be offered full, accurate, understandable and timely information about their condition, its prognosis, the treatment options, and the associated risks and benefits.' In addition, patients 'should also be offered understandable, time accurate, relevant information about the quality of care available to them in a particular NHS organisation, and how it compares with standards of good quality and performance elsewhere. This should include information about the outcomes of care, as well as information about other relevant aspects of quality, such as patients' experience.' Whenever possible, patients and their families 'should have a chance to take information away with them, to reflect upon information, and to ask questions. The Department also recognises that steps have to be taken to recognise and support patients for whom greater knowledge causes or increases anxiety and endorse the principle of support by encouraging patients to take another person with them to the consultation.'

Because of the content and context of the Kennedy Report, it is relatively light on patient responsibilities, but if patients have these resources, then they too have responsibilities and can participate and share in decision-making.

4.4.3 Shared decision-making

The Picker Institute, developed in Boston, is committed to measuring the experience of patients, rather than their degree of satisfaction, because:

- satisfaction is determined not only by the quality of the service but also by the expectations of the patient, whereas

- patient experience provides a direct measure of service quality.

What emerges from Picker Europe, for example through its work on the national survey of patients in the National Health Service, is that patients feel they are not sufficiently included in decision-making. This led a group based on Picker Europe to propose that shared decision-making should be an objective of clinical practice and healthcare. Shared decision-making, however, is only one element of patient-centred care, defined in a leader in the *British Medical Journal* as care which 'took into account the patient's desire for information and for sharing decision-making, and responding appropriately'.[23]

The *BMJ* editorial addressed three questions:

- do patients want it?

- do doctors practise it?

- what are its benefits?

4.4.3.1 Do patients want patient-centred care?

The study on which the *BMJ* editorial was based[24] found, like many other studies, that patients do want patient-centred care which:

explores the patient's main reason for the visit, [their] concerns and need for information;

seeks an integrated understanding of the patient's world – that is, their whole person, emotional needs and life issues;

finds common ground on what the problem is and mutually agrees management;

enhances prevention and health promotion;

enhances the continuing relationship between the patient and doctor.

Some patients want to understand fully and to be in control[25,26]; the majority want more control and involvement than they get at present.

4.4.3.2 Do clinicians practise it?

Because patient-centred care is a spectrum, it is hard to answer this question categorically. Almost all clinicians try to practise patient-centred care but with varying degrees of success, as perceived by the patient. Furthermore, many doctors now try to tailor their decision-making to take into account the patient's desire for patient-centred care and this is a difficult thing to do. One study found that the desire for a patient-centred approach with shared decision-making was highest in patients who were:

- worried,
- anxious or depressed,
- unemployed.

Patients who feel vulnerable want the doctor to focus on the whole person; those who have a clear diagnosis, and who are not anxious or depressed, also want to be at the centre of the clinician's attention but are willing to accept that the main focus should be on the disease.

4.4.3.3 Does it lead to a better outcome?

The answer is positive; patient-centred care is better for patients, clinicians and the health service.

Of central importance in delivering patient-centred care is good communication. This was reviewed at a conference in Toronto which came to the conclusion that:

- communication problems in medical practice are both important and common;

- the quality of clinical communication is related to positive health outcomes;

- beneficial clinical communication is feasible routinely in clinical practice and can be achieved during normal clinical encounters without unduly prolonging them;

- to become effective communicators, clinicians must master a set of skills, knowledge and attitudes.

Part of the problem lies in the language that people use, and a study of the language used in the consultation found that even when doctors were intending to practise patient-centred care and were committed to good communication, the medical jargon they used all too easily maintained the unfavourable power balance. It is not only medical terms such as 'cancer' which the patients need to understand, but also the grammar of clinical practice, and concepts such as 'risk' and 'effectiveness'.

Communication can be assisted by decision aids on paper, compact disc and on the World Wide Web and decision aids do improve knowledge and help patients be more active in decision-making without increasing their anxiety.

The clinician alone, no matter how well trained, may find it very difficult to communicate well but a health service cannot be run with leaflets and Web sites alone; human contact and interaction is of central importance in health care and will remain so. There have been calls for patients to be more responsible but what is needed is for patients to be allowed the opportunity to be resourceful. Suddenly the topic is hot, both politically and in the world of research, as shown in a separate supplement to the influential journal *Quality in Health Care*, published in 2001 with twelve papers commissioned by the Medical Research Council on 'Engaging Patients in Decisions.[27] We already have knowledge about both the methods and the benefits of engagement. What is needed is to get the knowledge into action. Clinicians need to be better communicators and more patient focused, but before planning more investment in professional education, priority should be given to developing resourceful patients.

References

(1)   Krishna, S., Bales, E.A., Spencer, D.C., Griffin, J.Z., and Boren, S.A. (1997) Clinical trials of interactive computerized patient education. *J. Family Practice*, 45: 25-33.

(2)   Chalmers, I. (2000) A patient's attitude to the use of research evidence for guiding individual choices and decisions in healthcare. *Clinical Risk*, 6: 227-230.

(3)   Gupta, K., Hooton, T.M., Roberts, P.L. and Stamm, W.E. (2001) Patient-initiated treatment of uncomplicated recurrent urinary tract infections in young women. *Ann. Intern. Med.*, 135: 9-16.

(4)   O'Connor, A. (2001) Using patient decision aids to promote evidence-based decision-making. *Evidence-based Medicine*, 6: 100-2.

(5)   van Wersch, A. and Eccles, M. (2001) Involvement of consumers in the development of evidence-based clinical guidelines: practical experiences from the North of England evidence-based guideline development programme. *Quality in Health Care*, 10: 10-16.

(6)   Coulter, A. (2001) Informed choice in screening. Special Issue of *Health Expectations*, Blackwells Science.

(7)   Walter, L.C. and Covinsky, K.E. (2001) Cancer screening in elderly patients. *JAMA*, 285: 2750-6.

(8)   Welch, H.G. (2001) Informed choice in cancer screening. *JAMA*, 285: 2776-8.

(9)   An organisation with a memory: report of an expert group on learning from adverse events in the NHS. (2000) Department of Health.

(10)   Richardson, W.C., Berwick, D.M., Bisgard, J.C., Bristow, L.R. et al. (2000) Preventing death and injury from medical errors requires dramatic system-wide changes. Institute of Medicine, Division of Health Care Studies.

(11)   Oliver, S., Rajan, L., Turner, H., Oakley, A., Entwistle, V., Watt, I., Sheldon, T.A. and Rosser, J. (1996) Informed choice for users of health services: views on ultrasonography leaflets of women in early pregnancy, midwives and ultrasonographers. *BMJ*, 313: 1251-5.

(12)   Degner, L.F., Kristjanson, L.J., Bowman, D., Sloan, J.A., Carriere, K.C., O'Neil, J., Bilodeau, B., Watson, P. and Mueller, B. (1997) Information needs and decisional preferences in women with breast cancer. *JAMA*, 277: 1485-92.

(13)   Braddock, C.H., Edwards, K.A., Hasenberg, N.M., Laidley, T.L. and Levinson, W. (1999) Informed Decision-Making in Outpatient Practice. Time to get back to basics. *JAMA*, 282: 2313-20.

(14)   Barry, M.J. (1999) Involving Patients in Medical Decisions. How Can Physicians Do Better? (Editorial) *JAMA*, 282: 2356-7.

(15)   Coulehan, J.L., Platt, F.W., Lin, C.T., Egener, B., Frankel, R., Lown, B. and Salazar, W.H. (2001) 'Let me see if I have this right...' Words that help build empathy. *Ann.Intern.Med.*, 135:221-7

(16)   Grant, M.D., Rudberg, M.A. and Brody, J.A. (1998) Gastrostomy

Placement and Mortality Among Hospitalized Medicare Beneficiaries. *JAMA,* 279:1973-5

(17) Gardner, K. and Chapple, A. (1999) Barriers to referral in patients with angina: qualitative study. *BMJ,* 319:418-20

(18) Oxman, A.D., Chalmers, I., and Sackett, D.L. (2001) A practical guide to informed consent to treatment. *BMJ,* 323:1464-6

(19) Smith, R. (2001) Why are doctors so unhappy? *BMJ,* 322: 1073-4.

(20) Mechanic, D. (2001) How should hamsters run? Some observations about sufficient patient time in primary care. *BMJ,* 323: 266-8.

(21) Rees, L. and Weil, A. (2001) Integrated medicine. *BMJ,* 322: 119-20.

(22) Platt, F.W. and Gaspar, D.L. (2001) Tell me about yourself: the patient-centered interview. *Ann. Intern. Med.,* 134: 1079-85.

(23) Stewart, M. (2001) Towards a global definition of patient centred care. *BMJ,* 322: 444-5.

(24) Little, P., Everitt, H., Williamson, I., Warner, G., et al. (2001) Preferences of patients for patient-centred approach to consultation in primary care: observational study. *BMJ,* 322: 468-72.

(25) Irwig, J., Irwig, L. and Sweet, M. (1999) *Smart Health Choices,* Churchill Livingstone.

(26) Oster, N., Thams, T. and Joseff, D. (2000) *Making informed medical decisions,* O'Reilly.

(27) Thomson, R., Bowling A. and Moss F. (2001) Engaging patients in decisions: a challenge to healthcare delivery and public health. *Quality in Health Care,* 10: Supplement 1.

THE RESOURCEFUL PATIENT TOOLKIT

The Resourceful Patient Web site www.resourcefulpatient.org contains resources and links to other sources of help for patients, clinicians and managers.

The resources or links to resources, available only on the Web site are:

- books for patients (quality assured books for patients);
- Web-based resources for clinicians and managers who want help to enable patients to become resourceful;
- the Bookshop of the Book;
- the instructive Advance Directive – a model Living Will for discussion and reflection;
- a programme to promote public understanding of the science and art of medicine – a proposal for action;
- the Bristol Inquiry – the recommendations of the inquiry into paediatric cardiac surgery in Bristol, and the government's response to these recommendations;
- all the key Department of Health papers;
- an e-consultation vignette for discussion and reflection;
- a case study of the methods that can be used to tailor evidence derived from the study of groups of patients to take into account the condition and values of the individual patient (aspirin after myocardial infarction).

Bibliography

Balint, M., _The Doctor, the Patient and his Illness_
Beck, Ulrich, _The Risk Society_
Berne, E., _Games People Play_
Berne, E., _What do you say after you say Hello?_
Chartier, R., _The Order of Books_
Farrell, J.G., _The Siege of Krishnapur_
Galbraith, J.K., _The New Industrial Estate_
Gould, S.J., _Adam's Navel_
Gray, J.A M., _Evidence-based Healthcare_
Greenhalgh, T., _Narrative Medicine_
Grisham, J., _The Rainmaker_
Groopman, J., _Second Opinions: Stories of intuition and choice in the changing world of medicine_
Halberstam, D., _The Best and the Brightest_
Irwig, J., Irwig, L., and Sweet, M., _Smart Health Choices: how to make informed health decisions_
James, P.D., _The Black Tower_
Johns, A., _The Nature of the Book_
Krause, E., _The Death of the Guilds: The state capitation and the decline of the professions, 1930 to the present day_
Murray, J.F., _Intensive Care: a Doctor's Journal_
Palmer, M., _The Patient_
Sackett D.L., Straus S.E., Richardson W.S., Rosenberg W. and Haynes R.B., _Evidence-based Medicine – How to Practice and Teach EBM_
Schama, S., _Landscape and Memory_
Shaw, G.B., _The Doctor's Dilemma_
Starr, Paul, _The Social Transformation of American Medicine_
The Oxford Textbook of Medicine
Usherwood, T., _Understanding the Consultation_
Van Allan, E.J., _You Decide_
Weil, A., _Spontaneous Healing_

Index

Colophon

This book is typeset in Gill Sans 10 on 11.5 point, and printed on 90gm Xerox Colotech; the cover is 280gm Xerox gloss coated Colotech.

It would not have been possible without:

Software

Adobe Acrobat, Adobe Illustrator, Adobe Photoshop, Macromedia Dreamweaver, Microsoft Word, Qualcomm Eudora, QuarkXPress

Hardware

Apple Macintosh G4, Canon EOS 500, Compaq iPAQs, Dell and Sony notebooks, Heidelberg Digimaster 9110, Hewlett-Packard Laserjets, Kolbus Ratio Binder, Umax Scanner, Xerox Docucolor 2060

People

Robert Hay, Steve Neville, Harry Rutter, Jo Wainwright